Transfusion Medicine
Step by Step
Technical Manual
of
Blood Components Preparation

A unit of whole blood can save four lives

Transfusion Medicine
Step by Step Technical Manual of Blood Components Preparation

A unit of whole blood can save four lives

Bibekananda Mukherjee
BSc DMLT WHO Fellow
Senior Technologist
Department of Transfusion Medicine
Bokaro General Hospital, Bokaro Steel Plant
Steel Authority of India Limited
Bokaro Steel city, Jharkhand, India

Forewords
K Ghosh
Utpal Chaudhuri
Sudipta Sekhar Das

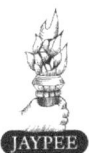

JAYPEE BROTHERS MEDICAL PUBLISHERS
The Health Sciences Publisher
New Delhi | London

Jaypee Brothers Medical Publishers (P) Ltd

Headquarters
EMCA House
23/23-B, Ansari Road, Daryaganj
New Delhi 110 002, India
Landline: +91-11-23272143,
+91-11-23272703
+91-11-23282021, +91-11-23245672
E-mail: jaypee@jaypeebrothers.com

Overseas Office
JP Medical Ltd.
83, Victoria Street, London
SW1H 0HW (UK)
Phone: +44-20 3170 8910
E-mail: info@jpmedpub.com

Corporate Office
Jaypee Brothers Medical Publishers (P) Ltd.
4838/24, Ansari Road, Daryaganj
New Delhi 110 002, India
Phone: +91-11-43574357
Fax: +91-11-43574314
E-mail: jaypee@jaypeebrothers.com

EU GPSR Authorised Representative
Logos Europe, 9 rue Nicolas Poussin
17000, La Rochelle, France
Phone: +33 (0) 6 67 93 73 78
E-mail: Contact@logoseurope.eu

Website: www.jaypeebrothers.com
Website: www.jaypeedigital.com

© 2016, Jaypee Brothers Medical Publishers

The views and opinions expressed in this book are solely those of the original contributor(s)/author(s) and do not necessarily represent those of editor(s) of the book.

All rights reserved. No part of this publication may be reproduced, stored or transmitted in any form or by any means, electronic, mechanical, photocopying, recording or otherwise, without the prior permission in writing of the publishers.

All brand names and product names used in this book are trade names, service marks, trademarks or registered trademarks of their respective owners. The publisher is not associated with any product or vendor mentioned in this book.

Medical knowledge and practice change constantly. This book is designed to provide accurate, authoritative information about the subject matter in question. However, readers are advised to check the most current information available on procedures included and check information from the manufacturer of each product to be administered, to verify the recommended dose, formula, method and duration of administration, adverse effects and contraindications. It is the responsibility of the practitioner to take all appropriate safety precautions. Neither the publisher nor the author(s)/editor(s) assume any liability for any injury and/or damage to persons or property arising from or related to use of material in this book.

This book is sold on the understanding that the publisher is not engaged in providing professional medical services. If such advice or services are required, the services of a competent medical professional should be sought.

Every effort has been made where necessary to contact holders of copyright to obtain permission to reproduce copyright material. If any have been inadvertently overlooked, the publisher will be pleased to make the necessary arrangements at the first opportunity.

Inquiries for bulk sales may be solicited at: jaypee@jaypeebrothers.com

Step by Step Technical Manual of Blood Components Preparation

First Edition: 2016, Reprint: 2023, **2025**

ISBN 978-93-5152-604-9

Printed in India

*Dedicated to
my respected father
Late Nonigopal Mukherjee
respected mother
Late Shankari Mukherjee
and
beloved brother
Late Ramkrishna Mukherjee (1968–2005)
whose inspirations have encouraged
me for this work*

Foreword

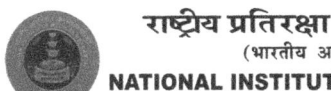

राष्ट्रीय प्रतिरक्षा रूधिर विज्ञान संस्थान
(भारतीय आयुर्विज्ञान अनुसंधान परिषद)
NATIONAL INSTITUTE OF IMMUNOHAEMATOLOGY
(INDIAN COUNCIL OF MEDICAL RESEARCH)

Dr Kanjaksha Ghosh
MD (Med), DNB (Haem.), FRC Path (Lond.), FACP (USA),
MRCP (Ire), MRCP (UK), FAMS, FNASc, FICP
Director &
Hon. Professor
Department of Hematology
KEM Hospital

D.O. No.:

Date:

It gives me immense pleasure and a sense of pride to see that our WHO trainee Bibekananda Mukherjee has written a small but very useful handbook detailing how blood components may be prepared in a blood bank. The book is well-illustrated, compact, full of figures for easy comprehension and can be easily carried in a small bag. In India, increasingly more and more medical colleges are coming up with curriculam of "MD" program in transfusion medicine. Similarly, trainee technicians for blood banks and transfusion medicine setups need to know in their fingertips how blood components can be produced and how its quality can be maintained. Mukherjee's book will fill up a long felt gap in this area. It will be useful to doctors and technicians alike, if they are in the field of transfusion medicine. I wish all the success for this book.

K GHOSH
Director
National Institute of
Immunohaematology (ICMR)
13th Floor, New Multistoreyed Bldg,
KEM Hospital Campus, Parel
Mumbai, Maharashtra

Foreword

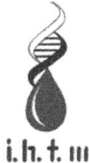

GOVERNMENT OF WEST BENGAL

Institute of Haematology & Transfusion Medicine

3rd floor, MCH Building

Medical College, Kolkata

88 College Street

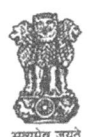

It is a great pleasure for me to write a foreword for the book *Step by Step Technical Manual of Blood Components Preparation* written by Bibekananda Mukherjee. The book is compact and well-illustrated. The pictorial demonstrations will help the students understand the procedures with ease. It will help not only the medical technologists working in blood banks but also to the postgraduate students of MD transfusion medicine. There was hardly any book in this subject that can help students and trainees in their day-to-day work. The book would help to fill up their this lacuna.

I wish all the success for this book.

Utpal Chaudhuri
Director, IHTM

Foreword

Dr Sudipta Sekhar Das
MD (Transfusion Medicine, SGPGIMS)
PDCC (Transfusion Medicine, SGPGIMS)
Consultant & Incharge, Department of
Transfusion Medicine
Associate Professor - AHERF
E-mail : sudipta.sgpgi@yahoo.co.in
Mobile : +91 96419 49552

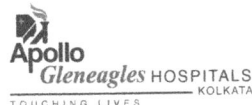 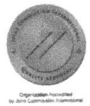

It gives me immense pleasure to mention the effort of Bibekananda Mukherjee who besides his busy working schedule managed to prepare this *Step by Step Technical Manual of Blood Components Preparation*. Mukherjee has very well enumerated his technical skill and experiences in this manual. Hope this technical manual would enable the blood bank professionals and other blood users to update their knowledge of blood component preparation methodology and use of blood and blood components in clinical practice.

With regards

Sudipta Sekhar Das

Preface

The extent to which human blood is used therapeutically demands that the quality and safety of whole blood components be ensured in order and primarily to prevent the transmission of diseases. Since 20 years of my technical association with blood bank of Bokaro General Hospital, I feel that care should be taken throughout the whole blood transfusion chain, starting from the collection, testing, component preparation, processing, and storage and also for safe distribution.

In our country today, the use of blood components remains an essential-step in therapy, and as a matter of fact, majority of blood bank and blood laboratories prepare blood components after receiving the whole blood. With over five years of practical experience in preparation of blood components in my blood bank, I feel that several technical tips are essential for qualitative preparation of blood components. Moreover, during my recent WHO fellowship training, I have acquired several technical know-how, which I feel to communicate to those who are engaged in such vital activities.

Writing of this technical manual is an attempt to help those young persons who are sincerely engaged in such profession. I have tried my best effort to present my practical knowledge regarding blood component preparation. The book covers all areas of the subject, i.e. selection of donors, safe handling of equipments, calibration, preparation of components, component storage, component thawing, issue of component, transfusion doses, quality control, etc. Many important informations are presented clearly for quality product, which are normally overlooked or escaped by an author. This manual meets the ready references for safe and qualitative preparation of blood components.

Bibekananda Mukherjee

Acknowledgments

I wish to thank all those working in department of Transfusion Medicine who have helped in the preparation of this technical manual and expressed their ideas regarding this book.

I am very much indebted to (Prof) Dr Kanjaksha Ghosh, Director NIIH (ICMR), Mumbai, who has motivated me for giving special attention for blood bank methodology and blood component preparation during my fellowship. I express my thanks because he spent his valuable time to read this manual and exporessed his fillings regarding the manual.

I am indebted to (Prof) Dr Utpal Chaudhuri, Director IHTM, Medical College Kolkata, West Bengal, India for his valuable recommendation regarding my book.

I am specially indebted to Dr Sudipta Sekhar Das, MD, PDCC (Transfusion Medicine SGPGIMS, Lucknow), Head of the Department of Transfusion Medicine, Apollo Gleneagles Hospital, Kolkata, West Bengal, India for giving me proper guidance to complete this work.

I express my gratitude to honorable Doctors, viz Dr Prasun Bhattacharya, MD (Transfusion Medicine), Assistant Professor and Head, Department of Immunohematology and Blood Transfusion, Medical College Kolkata; Dr B Bhattacharjee (Deputy Director, Tech) SBTC,WB and Ex-HOD (Transfusion Medicine), RG Kar Medical College; Dr Sidda Raju, Head, Department of Pathology, JIPMER Medical College, Puduchery; Dr Madhusudan Mandal, Head (Transfusion Medicine), National Medical College, Kolkata; Dr Dilip Panda, Head (Transfusion Medicine), NRS Medical College, Kolkata; Dr Subhasis Chakrabarty, Central Blood Bank (Institute of Immunohematology and Transfusion Medicine) Kolkata, Dr Tapan Kr Ghosh,

Head, Department of Pathology, BS Medical College and Hospital, Bankura (WB) and Dr Alok Kumar Mandal, Head, (Transfusion Medicine), BS Medical College and Hospital, Bankura (WB), and (Prof) Dr Malay Ghosh (WB), Director RBTC, RG Kar Medical College Kolkata (WB).

Dr Tushar Kanti Gupta, MO (Transfusion Medicine), AMRI Hospital Kolkata, Dr Akhil Kr Mandal, Ex-Director, Institute of Transfusion Medicine and Immunohaematology, Central Blood Bank, Kolkata, Dr Devashish R Desai, MO, Life Care Medical Complex, Kolkata, and Dr Prosanto Chowdhury, Member of Thalassemia International Federation, who have spent their valuable time to read this manual and expressed their feelings regarding the manual.

I am also indebted to Dr YP Bhattacharya and Dr GN Sahoo (DMS, BGH/BSL), Dr AK Singh, Director, I/C (BGH, BSL), Shri Biswarup Mukhopadhyay, GM, (HRD/BSL), Dr Mrs Manju Roy, Ex-HOD (BGH, Pathology), Dr Upendra Mohanty Ex-JD, Dr RN Pradhan JD, Dr KN Thakur JD, Dr TM Singh JD, Dr SK Sinha JD, Dr Prasanta Kumar Sarkar JD, Dr NK Das JD, Dr Subrato Dey JD, Dr Shrawan Kumar I/C (Transfusion Medicine), Dr Prakash Pandey, Dr Md Isha, Dr M Rajak, Dr Aninda Mandal, Dr Aniruddha Bandopadhyay, for their proper guidance and moral support.

I am indebted to Dr Trinath Pachal (BGH, BSL) Dr Mrs K Vasantha, Dr Ajit C Gorakshakar, Dr Mrs Swati Kulkarni (NIIH, ICMR Mumbai), Dr RK Verma and Mr Sanjay Chaudhary (Jamshedpur Blood Bank), Dr Arshad Hassan Siddiqie, Blood Bank Officer (Jammu and Kashmir, Health Department), Dr Sagar Chatterjee (Ortho Dign), Mr Sabyasachi Hazra, Mr Arunangshu Saha, and Production Unit (Kolkata branch) of M/s Jaypee Brothers Medical Publishers (P) Ltd., New Delhi, India and Mr Dhruba Mandal (IBTMI, Kolkata) for their valuable contribution in writing the manual.

I also want to acknowledge my elder brother respected Shri Swapan Kumar Mukhopadhyay, Mrs Jharna Mukherjee (Baudi), Mrs Mithu Banerjee (Didi), Mrs Reena Sarkar (Baudi), Dr Mrs Anju Parira, Shri Sushanta Chakraborty (Brother-in-law), Shri Rajarshi Mukherjee (Nephew), Shri Indranil Chakrabarty (nephew), Mr Sujit Kr Pal, Mr Subal Dutta, Mr Subhas Chandra Dey (Jamshedpur Blood Bank), Mr Avijit Pal (RSP, Hospital), Mr Pradeep Kr Ghosal and Mr Samarendra Kundu (Friend), Mr Avishek Kumar, Mr Animesh Mukherjee, Mr Jayanta Roy Chaudhary Mr Tapan Mohanta (Friend), Mr Angsuman Banerjee (Nephew), Miss Meghna Chatterjee (Cousin), Mrs Uma Unnikrishnan who always encourage and boost up me for good work.

Lastly, I express my thanks to my wife Mrs Anjali Mukherjee, daughter Miss Deep Shikha Mukherjee (Diya) and my best friend Mr Ghanshyam Sharma for helping and cooperating me for this book.

Contents

Chapter 1 : Introduction   **1**
- What is better—Whole blood or components? 1

Chapter 2 : Definition of Blood Components   **3**
- Functions of blood components 3

Chapter 3 : Blood Components Separation   **5**
- Introduction 5

Chapter 4 : Benefits and Advantages of Blood Components   **7**
- The following components are benefited 8

Chapter 5 : Methodology of Blood Components Preparation   **10**
- Donor selection 10
- Blood collection techniques for donor 11
- General awareness and precaution for donor 14
- Care after donation 15
- Health benefits of donating blood 17
- Defer the donor temporarily 18
- Restricted person for blood donation 19
- Blood group choice for blood and blood components 21
- ABO blood group systems 24
- Safe plasma transfusion 24
- Common blood type in Indian people 24
- Bag selection 25
- Selection of bag for donating blood 27
- Precautions required for blood components preparation area 28
- Precautions required for blood components preparation 30

- Common things to be done before preparation of blood components 31
- Common things to be done during preparation of blood components 35

Chapter 6 : Basic Informations for Blood Components Product   **37**
- Instruction followed for blood components preparation 37
- Materials required for blood components product 41

Chapter 7 : Safe Handling of Equipments   **44**
- Refrigerated centrifuge (Cryofuge 6000i) 45
- Programing of cryofuge 6000i 45
- Handling of cryofuge centrifuge 6000i and other models of refrigerated centrifuge 46
- Check calibration of cryofuge centrifuge 6000i and other models of refrigerated centrifuge 48
- Horizontal laminar airflow bench 53
- Circulating plasma/cryowater bath 54
- Handling of circulating plasma/cryowater bath 55
- Electronic sealer 55
- Operation of electronic sealer 55

Chapter 8 : Preparation of Blood Components Procedures   **57**
- Blood components preparation 57
- Packed red blood cell (PRBC)/fresh frozen plasma (FFP) by double bags collection 58
- Leuko-depleted packed cell/fresh frozen plasma by triple bags collection 63
- Packed red blood cell (PRBC)/cryoprecipitate/cryopoor plasma by triple bags collection 65
- Cryoprecipitate component preparation 66

- Packed red blood cell (PRBC)/platelets concentrate/platelets-poor plasma/Fresh frozen plasma (PPP/FFP) by random donor in triple bags collection 69
- Packed red blood cell (PRBC) (leuko-depleted)/platelets concentrate by (buffy-coat method)/FFP preparation in quadruple bags 71
- Instruction follows after preparation of platelet concentrate in triple bags and quadruple bags 74
- Leuko-depleted packed cell, FFP and cryoprecipitate component preparation by quadruple bags 78
- Packed red blood cell (leuko-depleted), fresh frozen plasma/cryoprecipitate by quadruple bags (SAGM-2/Adsol preservative) 81
- Packed red blood cell (leuko-depleted)/platelets concentrate by (PRP method) and platelet-poor plasma (PPP/ FFP) in quadruple bags 84
- Packed red blood cell (PRBC) /platelets concentrate by (PRP method)/platelet-poor plasma (PPP/FFP)/cryoprecipitate or required amount of FFP for pediatrics patient in quadruple bags 87
- Saline-washed packed red blood cell (PRBC) in double bags preparation (450 mL/350 mL) 90

Chapter 9 : Preservation and Distribution of Blood Components   **94**
- Storage of blood components 94

- Thawing procedure 94
- Procedure to issue components 96

Chapter 10 : Component Transfusion‰s Dose and Rate of Infusion — 98
- Fresh frozen plasma 98
- Platelets concentrate 99
- Cryoprecipitate 100
- Infusion rates of various components 102

Chapter 11 : Quality Control — 103
- Sterility tests 103
- Quality control specifications and procedures for blood components 104

Chapter 12 : Biomedical Waste Management — 108
- Biomedical waste 108
- Biomedical waste management in relation to blood banking activities 110
- Preparation of sodium hypochlorite solution 112

Chapter 13 : Disinfection Protocol — 113
- Procedure 113

Chapter 14 : Sterilization — 115
- Autoclave (sterilizer) 115

Chapter 15 : Blood Bank Refrigerator — 118

Further Reading — 121
Index — 123

Abbreviations

ACCL	:	Acceleration
ADSOL	:	Adenine saline glucose mannitol
AHF	:	Antihemophilic factor
BV	:	Blood volume
CPDA	:	Citrate/phosphate/dextrose/adenine
CPP	:	Cryopoor plasma
DECL	:	Deceleration
EDTA	:	Ethylenediaminetetraacetic acid
FFP	:	Fresh frozen plasma
HCT	:	Hematocrit
PC	:	Packed cell (PRBC)
PL	:	Platelet
PLTC	:	Platelet concentrate
PPP	:	Platelet-poor plasma
PRBC	:	Packed red blood cell
PRP	:	Platelet-rich plasma
RBC	:	Red blood cell
RCF	:	Relative centrifugal force
RPM	:	Rotation per minute
RT	:	Room temperature
SAGM	:	Saline, adenine, glucose, mannitol
TEMP	:	Temperature
UV	:	Ultraviolet
WBC	:	White blood cell
BBNO	:	Blood bank number
C	:	Centigrade
HRS	:	Hours
Vol	:	Volume

History of Blood Banking/Blood Transfusion Service (BTS)

Presently, we transfuse blood with the hope to cure someone. Modern humanity is very much successful in transfusion medicine. This success was not reached in a day or in years. The history behind this success was succeeded by many reported failures, but our physical, emotional, spiritual and our intelligence had overcome all this difficulties. With our best efforts, we archived a successful procedure for an efficient, safe, and uncomplicated transfusion technique.

In 1492, to save life of a Pope Innocent VIII, an attempt of blood treatment was made; he had to drink 3 healthy boy's blood. The result was—Both were died.

Before Harvey's description of circulation in 1628 a technique for artery to artery administration of blood was proposed by Libavious in 1615.

The first successful blood transfusion was made by Blundell approx 150 years ago.

A rational explanation for incompatibility and hemolytic transfusion reaction was given by Landsteiner. He also discovered ABO group in 1900 and Rh system in 1940.

Blood Storage

The concept of blood banking or blood storage was put in practice after discovery of sodium citrate—with donor lying next to the patient in 1917. An effort was made to improve banking of blood and to extend lifespan of blood (RBC) from 21 days (ACD) to 28 days (CPD) to 35 days (CPDA-1) to 42 days (SAGM solution—Saline, adenine, glucose, mannitol).

Serology

The complication of blood transfusion is transmission of syphilis, after that Australia antigen hepatitis B and HIV in 1980. For blood transfusion service a mandatory screening is required for 5 diseases, (HBV, HCV, HIV, malaria, and syphilis).

Present Situation

Nowadays, blood transfusion faces the interesting challenges. In developed countries, how blood service should be organized through high technology, with addition of AIDS which provoked a great heightened emphasis of safety.

In many instances, the problems like lack of component therapy, level of shortage and unsolved safety problems are perpetuated by financial limitations, endemic infections, and political instability.

Blood is needed for its lifesaving properties and cannot justify its provision with basic safety precaution is the fact, but there could not be a single solution to these problems. During 1990s and onwards, future technical advances are taking place, including computerization, recombinant DNA techniques as well as improvement of cell separation and test for transfusion transmissible infections and plasma apheresis.

Early Attempts

The first attempt for blood transfusion was experimented to Pope Innocent VIII who was in coma. The blood of three boys was infused through the mouth, and both were died.

More sophisticated research in blood transfusion began in 17th century with Harvey's experiment with circulation of blood. The experiment was successful in transfusion between animals but, on human, continues poor results.

On June 15, 1667 Dr Jean Baptiste Denys, an eminent physician of king Louis XIV of France was administrator of the first fully documented human blood transfusion. He transfused the blood of a sheep into a 15-year-old boy and a laborer; both were survived. Then he withstoods the allergic reaction. The second attempt of transfusion was on a Swedish, Baron Bonde. He received two transfusions, and in second, he died. After that Denys performed some transfusion with calf's blood on Antoine Mauroy. After the third transfusion he also died. According to Mauroy's death, it was later determined that the arsenic poison was responsible for Mauroy's death. Finally, this procedure was banned in 1670 that continued for next 150 years.

In 1674, Antonie van Leeuwenhoek discovered the platelets.

First recorded successful blood transfusion occurred in England in 1665.

Richard Lower, a physician, kept a dog alive by transfusion of blood from other dogs.

Clotting was the principal obstacle for transfusion of blood. In 1869, Braxton Hicks recommended sodium phosphate as a nontoxic anticoagulant, and this was first example of blood preservation research.

Karl Landsteiner in 1901 discovered the ABO blood groups. He explained the serious reactions that occur in humans as a result of incompatible transfusion, and he won the Nobel prize.

An unprecedented blood transfusion was achieved in 1914. Huston reported the use of sodium citrate and glucose as diluents and anticoagulant solution for transfusion.

In 1915 minimum sodium citrate was used by Richard Lewishon to prevent clotting of blood, and this discovery opened the process of collection of blood from donors and to be stored for later transfusion to patient.

Rous and Turner introduced citrate-dextrose solution in 1916. Transfusion became more practical and safer for the patient from that time.

Early in 1932, the first blood bank was established in Leningrad Hospital, Russia to combat blood loss in World War II.

Dr Charles Drew was the pioneer to describe the techniques in blood transfusion and establishment of blood bank. Dr Drew was the first Director of first American red cross blood bank.

1939/40	: The Rh blood group system was discovered by Karl Landsteiner.
1940	: Edwin Cohn developed fractionation—plasma, albumin, protein.
1943	: P. Beeson published description of transfusion transmitted hepatitis.
1945	: Coombs, MouranT, and Race described the use of antihuman globulin.
1948	: Development of plastic bag for blood collection
1962	: Antihemophilic factor was discovered and use of component was understood.
1964	: Plasmapheresis introduced.
1965	: Cryoprecipitate was first used.
1971	: HBsAg antigen testing introduced for safe blood transfusion.
1981	: First AIDS case reported.
1985	: Screening of HIV in donated blood started.
1998	: Hepatitis C testing became mandatory for blood transfusion.

Plate 1

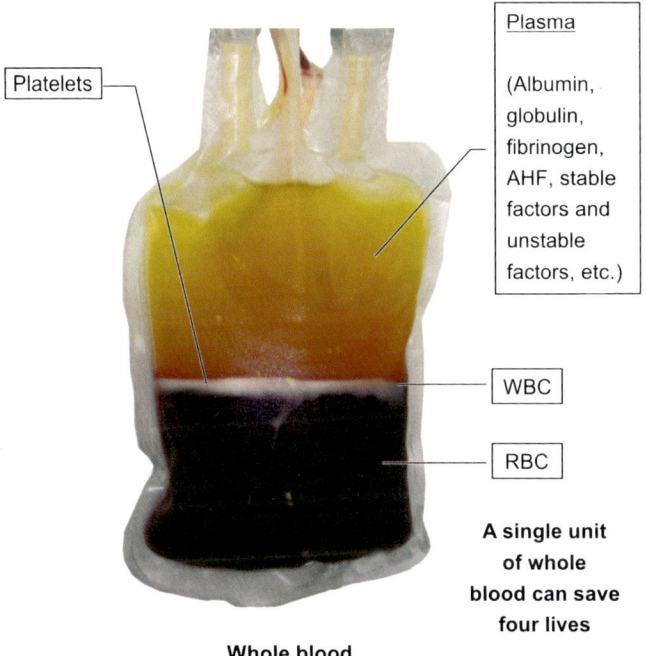

Figure 2.1: Whole blood

Plate 2

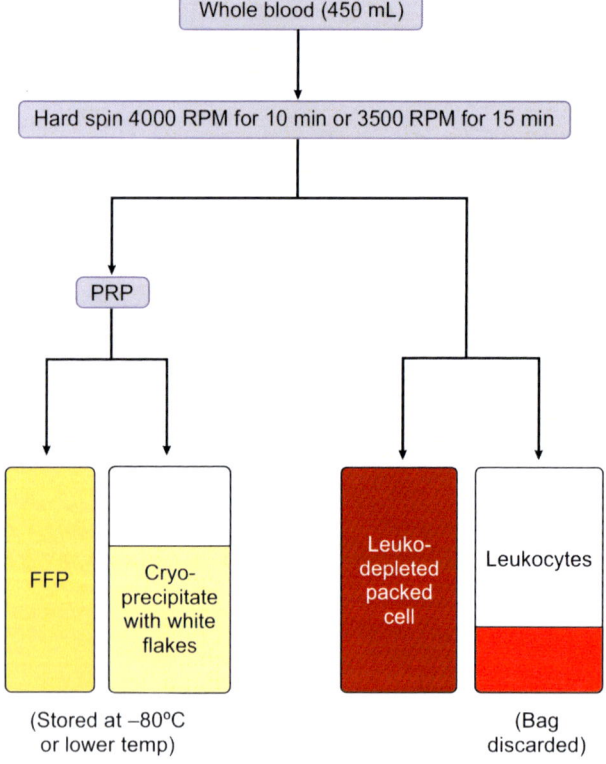

Flowchart 8.2: Blood components preparation by quadruple bags

Plate 3

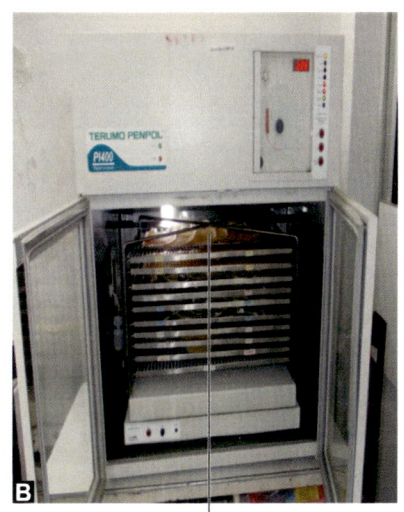

PLTC bags

Figure 8.5B: Platelet agitator incubator

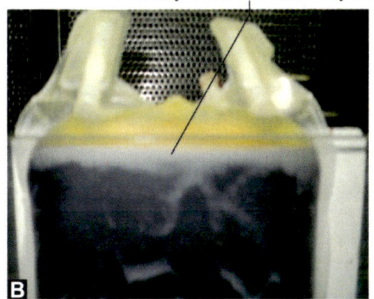

Buffy-coat with leukocytes

Figure 8.6B: Buffy-coat with leukocytes

Plate 4

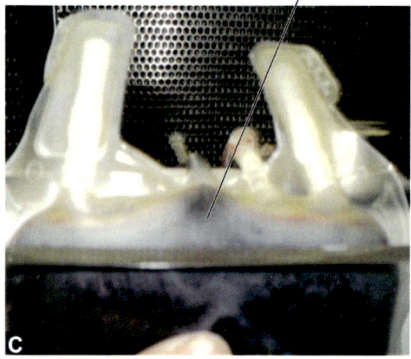

Figure 8.6C: Leukocytes coming out

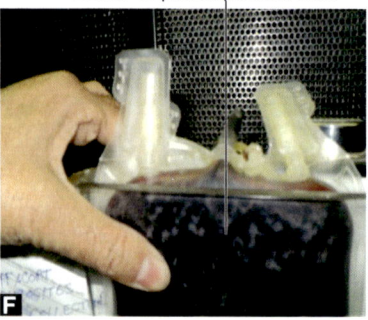

Figure 8.6F: Leuko-depleted packed cells

Plate 5

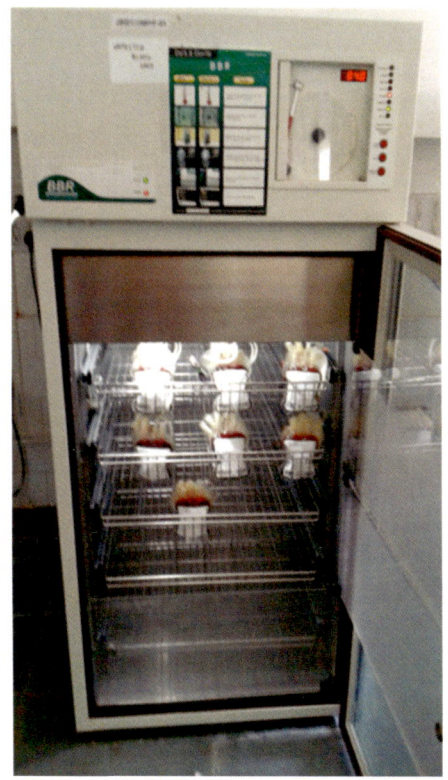

Figure 15.1: Blood bank refrigerator

Introduction

Chapter 1

In this world there is still no alternative of human blood. Scientist still cannot succeed in preparing synthetic blood or artificial blood. The amount of blood in a human body varies, depending on factors such as age, sex, overall health and even where a person lives. Scientists estimate the volume of blood in human body to be approximately 7% of body weight. **An average person has 5 6 liters of blood in the body. Blood is the fluid circulating the heart, arteries, capillaries, and veins; carrying nutrients and oxygen to body cells, and removing waste products and carbon dioxide**. So human beings are to be treated by only human blood. Today human blood is transfused in several ways and acts as medicine for treating a number of diseases. Components in a unit of whole blood include red blood cells, white blood cells, plasma, and platelets. Human blood consists of 55% plasma, 45% RBC, 0.1% WBC, and 0.17% platelets (See Fig. 2.1).

What is Better—Whole Blood or Components?

In our body there is 60–80 mL blood/kg of body weight. From this 16 mL is reserved. For donating of blood, the international prescribed standards says that a healthy person donates 8 mL/kg body weight of blood. Blood bags are available only in 350 mL and 450 mL size. So a person whose weight is above 45 kg can donate only 350 mL of blood, when the person whose weight is above 55 kg can donate 450 mL of blood. Whole blood is commonly obtained through blood donation and can be transfused directly or broken down into blood components that can be transfused separately.

Two methods are applied for preparation of components. One is the apheresis methodology, where a particular component is harvested from the donor by an automated machine. And another is whole blood collected from a healthy donor by aseptic means. Each whole blood is then processed to prepare various components.

With the availability of blood component preparation methodology now more than one patient is benefited from a unit of whole blood. For example the packed red blood cell can be transfused to thalassemia patients and the plasma and platelet can be issued to patients suffering from coagulopathy and dengue respectively. For thrombocytopenia cases platelets concentrate is more beneficial. Such patient should always receive a complete hemostatic dose of platelet which may comprise of 4–6 units platelet concentrates as per body weight. Blood banking involves collection, preparation, storage, and issue of blood and blood components after compatibility testing.

Definition of Blood Components

Chapter 2

Blood component therapy is also called blood transfusion. Blood components are various parts of blood like red blood cells (RBCs), platelets, granulocytes, and plasma. Separated from one another by conventional blood bank method by centrifugation because of their different specific gravities, different centrifugal force, different time, and different temperature change according to needs.

1. **Cellular components**: RBCs or packed cells, leukocyte-depleted red cells, platelets concentrate, platelet apheresis, leukocytes-depleted platelet concentrate.
2. **Noncellular plasma components**: Fresh frozen plasma, cryoprecipitate, and cryopoor plasma.

Functions of Blood Components

- **RBC**: It supplies oxygen to different parts of the body and carries carbon dioxide and other waste products (Fig. 2.1).
- **WBC**: It fights/prevents infections of diseases. White blood cells (WBCs) producing antibodies to develop immunity against infections (Fig. 2.1 and See Figs 8.6B and C).
- **Plasma**: It is the liquid part of blood, composed of about 92% water, 7% vital proteins such as albumin, gamma globulin, antihemophilic factor, and other clotting factors, and 1% mineral salts, sugars, fats, hormones and vitamins (Fig. 2.1; See Plate 1 for color figure).

4 Step by Step Technical Manual of Blood Components Preparation

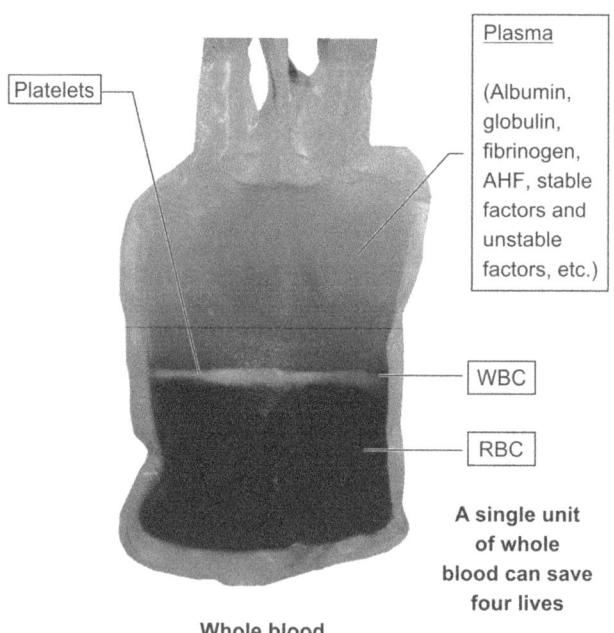

Figure 2.1: Whole blood

- **Platelets**: Platelets are produced in the bone marrow. The function of platelets is to prevent bleeding (important for blood clotting) (Fig. 2.1 and See Fig. 8.5B).

Blood Components Separation

Chapter 3

Introduction

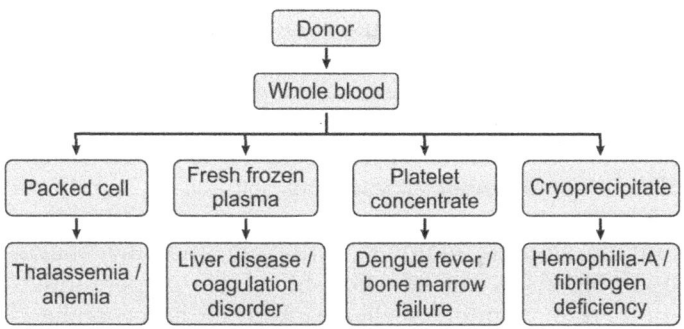

The blood components separation through whole blood is very useful contribution for modern medical practice. It also can reduce shortage of blood products. The advantage lies in the fact that, one unit of whole blood can now be utilized for more than one patient, the only appropriate component of the blood being used up by the patients as per their needs, thus not wasting the other important components which may be conserved for the other patients. **THUS, A SINGLE UNIT OF WHOLE BLOOD CAN SAVE FOUR LIVES**.

Thus, one can well-compensated with the acute shortage of blood units in growing developing countries, as far as the demand and supply of blood units is concerned because of the poor awareness of the blood donations.

Excess plasma available in a unit of whole blood is not beneficial for treatment of anemia; instead it causes volume overload, cardiac, and respiratory complications. Due to excess leukocytes in a blood unit patient may suffer from transfusion reaction like chill, fever, rigor, etc. **Usage of fresh whole blood refrigerated (2°C 6°C) has no significance in practical field.** Whole blood is rarely transfused, it happens only in cases of active blood loss like PPH bleeding (postpartum hemorrhage), accidental trauma for massive transfusion, patients with advanced renal or hepatic disease and in newborn baby exchange transfusion done for hyperbilirubinemia (blood stored for less than five days) whole blood transfusion can be considered. Neonates should not be transfused with whole blood/plasma component containing clinically significant antibodies. Plasma which is the liquid portion of the blood contains albumin, globulin, fibrinogen, and other coagulation factors. A unit of whole blood can prepare different types of components like packed cell/leuko-depleted packed cell, fresh frozen plasma, platelets concentrate, cryoprecipitate, etc.

Chapter 4

Benefits and Advantages of Blood Components

- In modern transfusion medicine, there is no use of whole blood. Blood is separated into components maximize the use of whole blood at present. When the blood components are separated all the important parts of blood can be used in whole blood. Platelets die and clotting factors become ineffective, and the patient, receives unwanted and ineffective components. There is no entity like fresh blood as the components have longer shelf life and the particular component deficit can be corrected in time with maximum utility and with minimum side effects.
- Maximizes the use of 1 unit of blood. Components can reduce the shortage of blood products. Components have greater shelf life than whole blood.
- The required components can give maximum benefit to a patient with minimum risk.
- Better proper patient management with appropriate deficient parts.
- Reduce risk of transfusion transmitted disease as well-adverse reaction of blood transfusion.
- Cost-effective product, from a unit of whole blood can prepare different types of components and supply according to patients' needs and cost-benefit goes to blood bank.
- Antigen is not present in plasma component product and Rh-factor need not to be considered, so Rh-negative person can receive Rh-positive plasma. But

Rh-positive plasma should not be given to Rh-negative women in reproductive age group.
- If ABO compatible plasma is unavailable then 'AB' group plasma can be transfused provided other alloantibodies are absent. 'AB' group plasma is also called 'neutral plasma'. It has no natural occurring antibodies.
- Usage of whole blood has no significance in practical field because stable factors and labile factors are reduced within 8 hours of storage at 2–6°C temperature except albumin and globulin.

The Following Components are Benefited

- **Packed red blood cell/leuko-depleted packed cell and saline-washed packed red cell**: These are very useful in anemic cases, like thalassemia, sickle cell anemia, hemolytic anemia, iron-deficiency anemia, etc. But SAGM-2 preservative packed cell should not be transfused below 12-year-old child and in old cases, as well as in renal failure cases, because mannitol may cause renal failure in those cases. So it is better to avoid that blood.
- **Leuko-depleted packed cell is very useful in these cases like chronic renal failure, malignancy, and multitransfusion**. Saline-washed red blood cell (RBC) is very useful for thalassemia patients. Because leukocytes are reduced by saline-washed as much as possible (See Figs 8.6E and F).
- **Fresh frozen plasma (FFP)**: One unit of FFP or thawed plasma is the plasma taken from a unit of whole blood. **FFP contains all coagulation factors (stable and unstable factors) in normal concentration like fibrinogen, factor-V, VII, VIII, X, XIII, etc. except platelets**. Plasma transfusion is indicated in patients with documented coagulation factor deficiencies and active bleeding or massive replacement with red blood

cells. It is also useful for burn cases, septicemia, liver diseases, etc. It must be ABO compatible. One unit of FFP is approximately 250 mL (See Fig. 8.2B).
- **Platelets concentrate:** Platelets are essential for the hemostasis. Platelets concentrate also contain about 50–60 mL plasma and small numbers of red blood cells and leukocytes. Platelet units must be maintained at 22°C and agitated during storage. It prevents bleeding due to thrombocytopenia. Conditions that may affect platelet function included renal failure, medications, leukemias, and congenital disorders. **It is also very useful for dengue fever, snake bite, etc.** (See Fig. 8.5B).

Pooled platelet concentrates are prepared by many centers by buffy-coat (6–8 units) pooling of same ABO type. If ABO-compatible platelets are unavailable, ABO-incompatible platelets can be substituted in adult patients, however all pediatric patients should preferably be transfused ABO-compatible platelets.

Contraindications

Not generally indicated for prophylaxis of bleeding in surgical patients, unless known to have significant preoperative platelet deficiency.
- **Platelet-rich plasma (PRP): A single unit of platelet-rich plasma is not beneficial for patients‰ treatment because amount of platelets is available very less in this bag.** Excess volume of plasma is harmful and carries other complications like volume overload or respiratory or cardiac problems.
- **Cryoprecipitate:** It is prepared from fresh frozen plasma and contains fibrinogen von Willebrand factor, factor VIII (very large amount) and fibronectin. Each unit from separate donor is suspended in 15–20 mL plasma, prior to pooling. Cryoprecipitate is helpful for hemophilia A, fibrinogen deficiency and von Willebrand disease.

Methodology of Blood Components Preparation

Chapter 5

Donor Selection

As donor selection is the most important and preliminary steps of blood banking service, blood must be collected from healthy, nonremunerated and safe donors to avoid any unwanted effects of the recipient.

Donor selection is done, based on the selection criteria described below.

- The interval between blood donations should be no less than 3 months.
- For platelet apheresis donation, interval time is 7 days.
- Nowaday's apheresis is becoming popular to maximize the use of blood, but in case of apheresis, donor deferral is different from conventional, e.g. if a donor donates blood in conventional method the donation interval is 3 months in male whereas if a donor donates plasma or platelet by apheresis method he can donate whole blood after 72 hours.
- The donor shall be in good health, mentally alert, and physically fit but a person having multiple sex partners, males having sex with males or a drug-addict/chronic alcoholic should not donate blood.
- The donor should be in the age group of 18–65 years.
- The donor should not be less than 45 kg for donation of 350 mL of blood (a donor can donate blood 8–9 mL/kg body weight).

- Hemoglobin should not be less than 12.5 gm/dL.
- The donor should be free from acute respiratory diseases.
- The donor should be free from any skin diseases at the site of phlebotomy.
- The arms and forearms of the donor should be free from skin punctures or scars indicative of professional blood donors or addiction of self-injected narcotics.
- Vein selection is very important for blood component products; it should flow freely by a clean single vein puncture.
- The blood pressure, pulse, and temperature should be within acceptable limits:
  - Systolic blood pressure not > 160 mmHg.
  - Diastolic pressure not > 90 mmHg.
  - Pulse regular, between 60 and 100 beats/minute.
  - Oral temperature 37.5°C +/− 0.2°C (98.6°F =/− 0.5°F)

  Systemic examination: Liver and spleen should not be palpable. There should not be any abnormality in heart or lungs.

Blood Collection Techniques for Donor

Blood donation should be carried out with the supervision of doctor (transfusion medicine or trained doctor), skilled trained technicians and nurse to insure a successful blood donation.

The life cycle of red blood cell is approximately 120 days. For healthy adults it is safe to donate blood, but after two donations it advised to have a gap of 3 months to regain the normal hemoglobin level of blood.

Phlebotomy Procedure

Important points:
1. Donor may be lying down with a pillow under head (in blood donation camp) or reclining in a comfortable

donor's couch/chair (in house collection), loosen tight garments.
2. All relevant records like donor's name, bag number, pilot tube number and name must be registered properly in the donor's card. The number on the blood bag and pilot test tubes must tally with donor's card.
3. The blood bag should be thoroughly examined for leaks, cracks or punctures. The anticoagulants must be inspected and it should be clear.

   The bag is to be kept over biomixer or with spring balance or on a blood bag weighing machine.
4. Apply BP cuff on donor's arm.
5. Should locate a vein 100%.
6. For puncture of vein, a prominent one has to be chosen.
7. The median cubital vein inside the elbow which is close to the skin is chosen for blood donation (Fig. 5.1).
8. Choose a healthy vein that doesn't rupture.
9. Access that vein without any injury.
10. Clean the vein area using alcohol, iodine then alcohol and dry the area.
11. The quality of the needle of the bag should be very good (ISO 3826), remove the plastic cover on the phlebotomy needle and perform venipuncture immediately.
12. The collection bag should be conducted with plastic tube and attached with needle. The needle should be inserted gently to the vein to collect the blood.
13. Advice the donor to continuously squeeze the hand roller to improve the blood flow.
14. When the bag is filled with blood the BP cuff is released and the needle is removed gently from donor's vein.
    A bandage is placed for the next few hours.

15. The blood line is clamped at two sites close to the donor side and cut in the middle.
16. Blood is collected in the pilot tubes from tubing, so that blood flows directly from donor's arm.
17. Donation time is approximately 5–10 minutes.

Dr James Blundell, a British Obstetrician made the first blood transfusion of human blood in 1818 for the treatment of postpartum hemorrhage (PPH).

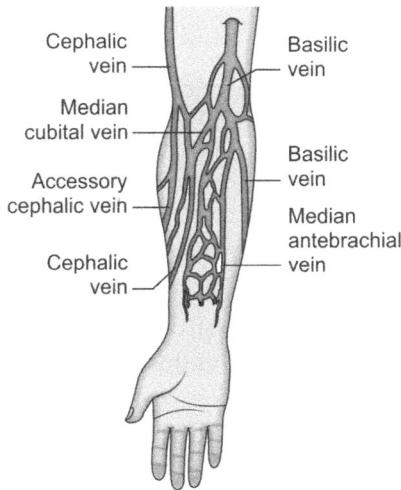

Figure 5.1: Median cubital vein inside the elbow

The median cubital vein inside the elbow which is close to the skin is chosen for blood donation.

| An average healthy person has 5–6 L of blood in the body | Dr James Blundell, a British Obstetrician made the first blood transfusion of human blood in 1818 for the treatment of postpartum hemorrhage (PPH) | Always wear gloves while handling blood specimens |

General Awareness and Precaution for Donor

Blood donation is a great contribution to our society. It is safe for human life. Only a healthy person can donate blood, because source of various infections comes through blood. Blood donation is carried out under the supervision of doctor (transfusion medicine or trained doctor), trained skilled technicians and nurse. Our mission is to donate better quality of blood and get good health.

Some important recommendations before and during donation of blood.

1. Before donation fill up a donor registration form and write answers very carefully.
2. If you have come from a long drive, take rest for at least 30 minutes and then donate blood.
3. Don't give blood with an empty stomach.
4. Eat a well-balanced diet including plenty of fluids before blood donation.
5. Don't open shoes before sitting on donor couch/chair. If you tie up shoelace after donation, blood may come out from bleeding point.
6. Only loose dress should be worn at the time of donating blood.
7. No pressure creating external device/thread should be in forearm of the donor from which blood is being drawn.
8. During donation of blood relax, listen to music and talk to other donors or technical staff (Fig. 5.2).
9. Donor must be kept under strict observation during and after donation.
10. Rest on the donor couch /chair for at least 10 minutes after the donation is completed and take permission to get up from donor couch/chair.

11. For vasovagal syndrome—The feet to be raised, clothing's to be loosen and belt to be removed.
    a. Give cold compress over forehead and back.
    b. Airway adequate.
    c. In vomiting turn the face to one side.
    d. Apply medicines accordingly (under the supervision of doctor).
12. During donation, if donor faints, stop blood collection immediately. Put the head at the end of the couch/chair down or alternatively raise the donor legs. Donor head may be placed between knees, fold both the legs and take aromatic ammonia spirit cotton just near the nose. Monitor blood pressure, pulse rate and temperature under the supervision of doctor (transfusion medicine or trained doctor).
13. Aromatic ammonia spirit is used to prevent or treat fainting.
14. Before starting collection of blood from donor, check routinely oxygen cylinder and emergency drugs as per directions of drugs and cosmetics rule.

Care After Donation

After blood donation the blood donor should be kept under observation and some advices must be given.

Immediately the following incident may occur after blood donation like syncope, vomiting, hyperventilation, and neuromuscular excitability like tetany, vasovagal reaction and bradycardia/hypotension. Rarely delayed syncope may occur 30 minutes – 1 hour after donation. The donors need to be observed after collection of blood, in order to attend any adverse reactions in the immediate postdonation period. Medical officer should attend the donor. The donor should report if any feeling of dizziness, vomiting, blackening, giddiness apart from these there may be local hematoma. So the phlebotomy site must be examined.

1. Take a rest for minimum of 20 minutes. Don't drive any vehicle after donation of blood.
2. Take some snacks and juice. It contains a high sugar and helps in backup of blood sugar.
3. Have a meal that contains high protein such as chicken, fish, egg, etc.
4. Don't take any kind of alcohol for 8–10 hours after donating the blood.
5. Don't do heavy work, i.e. jogging, gym, dancing, carrying heavy goods, etc.

How to relieve during donation of blood?

When you are donating blood, be relaxed and take deep breathe. Don't concentrate your mind to the process of donating blood. Listen to music or watch TV program.

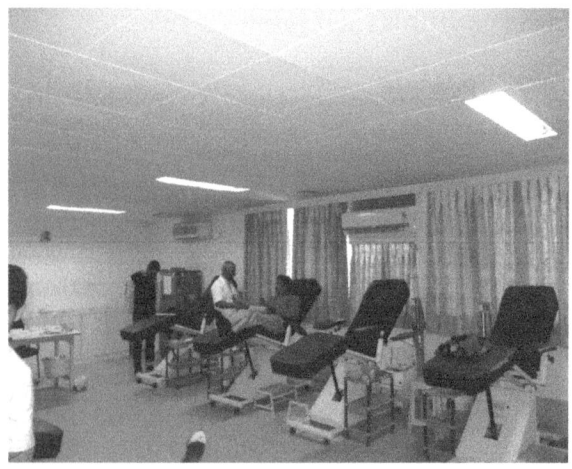

Figure 5.2: Blood donation room (safe donor), donating blood

Health Benefits of Donating Blood

Reduce the chance of heart diseases

- Reduce the one-third of chance of heart diseases as frequent donations reduce the accumulated and unwanted iron load from the body.
- Upon donation, donors are tested for syphilis, HIV, hepatitis, and other diseases.
- The reduction of accumulated iron in the body reduces the risk of cancer.
- Frequent donation of blood reduces the viscosity of blood.
- One unit of blood (450 mL) when donated burns 650 calories in donor's body so it helps in utilizing the calories.
- Blood donations helps in the formation of new RBC within 48 hours. After donating blood, the count of blood cells decreases in our body, which stimulates the bone marrow to produce new red blood cells in order to replenish the loss. So, it stimulates the production of new blood cells and refreshes the system.
- Moreover blood donation gives pleasure of saving someone's life.

> The average life cycle of a red blood cell is 120 days

> Have some rest minimum of 20 minutes after donation. Do not drive after donation of blood

Defer the Donor Temporarily

Defer the donor for the period mentioned as indicated in the Table 5.1.

Table 5.1: Defer the donor temporarily

Conditions	Period of deferment
Abortion	6 months
History of blood transfusion	6 months
Major surgery	12 months
Minor surgery	6 months
Typhoid	12 months after recovery
History of malaria and duly treated	3 months (endemic) and 3 years (nonendemic area)
Tattoo, ear puncture, acupuncture	6 months
Breastfeeding	12 months after delivery
Immunization (cholera, typhoid, diphtheria, tetanus, plague, gamma globulin)	15 days
Rabies vaccination	1 year after vaccination
Hepatitis in family or close contact	12 months
Hepatitis immune globulin	12 months
Chickenpox and mumps	3 weeks after recovery
Tuberculosis	5 years after complete treatment
Jaundice	12 months
Acute renal failure	5 years after treatment
Fever	15 days after recovery

Restricted Person for Blood Donation

Defer the donor permanently if suffering from any of the following diseases:
- Cancer
- Heart disease
- Abnormal bleeding tendencies
- Diabetes—Controlled on insulin
- Hepatitis B and C infections
- Chronic nephritis
- Asthma
- Epilepsy
- Leprosy
- Schizophrenia
- Endocrine disorders
- Kala-azar
- Cerebrovascular diseases
- Recipients of growth hormones or factor VIII conc.

> Blood is the fluid circulating in the heart, arteries, capillaries, and veins, carrying nutrients and oxygen to body cells, and removing waste products and carbon dioxide

Donors are permanently deferred if there are any signs or symptoms suggestive of AIDS

- History of high-risk behavior.
- Unexplained fever with night sweats for more than 1 month.
- Unexplained weight loss defined as 4.5 kg or more in 1 month.
- Swollen glands.
- Diarrhea.
- Kaposi's sarcoma.

Obtain informed consent of the donor

- Inform the donor regarding process of blood donation, risk associated, information regarding transfusion transmitted infection (TTI) screening, component preparation, and prior to donation.
- Ask the donor if he/she wants to be notified of the abnormal results of TTI screening.
- Obtain written consent on the blood donor registration card (for illiterate donors, thumb impression may be obtained).

Generation of donor registration (blood unit number) number

- If the donor meets the selection criteria, accept the donor for blood donation.
- Designate specific donors registration number.
- Enter the number on the donor's registration form, and request the donor to wait for phlebotomy.

> For optimum quality component preparation whole blood required is 450 mL because optimum platelets yields and other coagulation factors yields are more available there

> Cleanse the site for bleeding using alcohol, iodine then alcohol. Dry the site

Blood Group Choice for Blood and Blood Components (Tables 5.2 to 5.4)

Table 5.2: Blood group choice for PRBC and whole blood

Recipient	For Packed Red Blood Cells (PRBC)/ Whole Blood					
	Donor					
	A	B	O	AB	Rh-positive	Rh-negative
A	Option-I		Option-II			
B		Option-I	Option-II			
O			Option-I (the only option)			
AB		Option-II	Option-III	Option-I		
Rh-positive					Option-I	Option-II
Rh-negative						Option-I

* Rh-positive PRBC can be transferred to Rh-negative patient (postmenopausal females, old men) as a lifesaving measure and that to with consent from the patient or his relative and the treating physician once in a life.

Table 5.3: Blood group choice for PLTC

Recipient	For Platelet Concentrate (PLTC) Donor					
	A	B	O	AB	Rh-positive	Rh-negative
A	Option-I		Option-III	Option-II		
B		Option-I	Option-III	Option-II		
O	Option-III	Option-II	Option-I	Option-IV		
AB	Option-III	Option-II	Option-IV	Option-I		
Rh-positive					Option-I	Option-II
Rh-negative						Option-I

*Rh-positive platelets can be transferred to Rh-negative patient (postmenopausal females, old men) as a lifesaving measure and that to with consent from the patient or his relative and the treating physician as platelet has no antigen.

Table 5.4: Blood group choice for FFP

For Fresh Frozen Plasma (FFP) and Single Donor Plasma (SDP)						
Recipient	Donor					
	A	B	O	AB	Rh-positive	Rh-negative
A	Option-I			Option-II		
B		Option-I		Option-II		
O	Option-III	Option-II	Option-I	Option-IV		
AB				Option-I		
Rh-positive					Option-I	Option-II
Rh-negative					Option-II	Option-I

Methodology of Blood Components Preparation

ABO Blood Group Systems (Table 5.5)

Table 5.5: ABO blood group systems

The ABO Antigens and Corresponding Antibodies		
Antigen on RBC	Antibody in plasma/serum	Blood group
A	Anti-B	A
B	Anti-A	B
AB	None	AB
None	Anti-A and Anti-B	O

- **O** group has antibody but no antigen.
- **AB** group has antigen but no antibody.

> If ABO compatible plasma is unavailable then 'AB' group plasma can be transfused provided other alloantibodies are absent. 'AB' group plasma is also called neutral plasma

Safe Plasma Transfusion

- People with type '**O**' blood can get any type of plasma.
- People with type '**A**' blood can get 'A' or 'AB' plasma.
- People with type '**B**' blood can get 'B' or 'AB' plasma.
- People with type '**AB**' blood can get only 'AB' plasma.

Common Blood Type in Indian People

- O Rh-positive—36.5 %
- O Rh-negative—2.0 %
- A Rh-positive—22.1 %
- A Rh-negative—0.8 %
- B Rh-positive—30.9 %
- B Rh-negative—1.1 %
- AB Rh-positive—6.4 %
- AB Rh-negative—0.2 %

> In 1900, Landsteiner discovered ABO groups, Rh system was discovered in 1940 (Landsteiner)

> People with type 'AB' blood can get only 'AB' plasma

> Rh-positive platelets can be transferred to Rh-negative patient (postmenopausal females, old men) as a lifesaving measure and that to with consent from the patient or his relative and the treating physician as platelet has no antigen

> Rh-positive PRBC can be transferred to Rh-negative patient (postmenopausal females, old men) as a lifesaving measure and that to with consent from the patient or his relative and the treating physician once in a life

Bag Selection

- For blood component preparation, bag selection is very important.
- In blood bank 4 types of bags are used, viz. single, double, triple, and quadruple bags.
- Collect 450 mL of blood in triple bags and quadruple bags, and also collect 350 mL of blood in single bag and double bags. Some manufacturers make triple bags for 350 mL of blood collection and collect 450 mL of blood in double bags.
- Collect 350 mL of blood in single bag, and the single bag is used for whole blood. In this bag 49 mL CPDA preservatives are available. Life of the blood is 35 days.
- Collect 350 mL of blood in double bags, and the double bags are used for component preparation packed cells and fresh frozen plasma. In this bag 49 mL CPDA preservatives are available and life of the blood is 35 days.
- For preparation of FFP, PRBC, random donor's platelets collect 350 mL/450 mL of blood in the anticoagulated bag of triple bags, the satellite bags are used for the

preparation of FFP and random donor's platelets. The half-life period of PRBC depends on the anticoagulant present in the bag.
- Collect 350 mL/450 mL of blood in anticoagulant containing primary bag of quadruple bags. The quadruple bags are used for all types of components preparation like packed red blood cells/leuko-depleted packed red blood cell/FFP/platelets concentrate and cryoprecipitate. The ratio of CPDA-1 and blood is –14 mL of CPDA-1 for 100 mL of blood.
- Nowadays in addition 78 mL SAGM-2 preservatives for 350 mL of triple bag and 100 mL SAGM-2 preservatives for 450 mL of quadruple bag. Either triple or quadruple bag. If SAGM-2 is used of preservative the red cell life span is 42 days. In quadruple/triple bags one satellite bag is specially made for platelet concentrate preparation (Fig. 5.4).

Selection of bag for donating blood (Table 5.6)

Table 5.6: Selection of bag for donating blood

Donor		Components	Bags	
Weight	Aspirin intake	Required	Type	Qty. (mL) of blood
> 55 kg	No	PC+FFP+PLT	Triple or quadruple	450 mL
> 55 kg	Yes	PC+FFP PC+FVIIID+CRYO	Double	350/450 mL
45–55 kg	No	PC+FFP PC+FVIID+CRYO PC-PLT	Double	350 mL
45–55 kg	Yes	PC+FFP PC+FVIIID PC+FVIID+ CRYO	Double	350 mL

PC: Packed Cells, FFP: Fresh Frozen Plasma, PLT: Platelets, FVIIID: Factor VIII Deficient Plasma Cryo: Cryoprecipitate

Healthy person may donate 8 mL per kg body weight of blood

For blood components preparation after collection of blood, keep at room temperature (20°C–24°C) till processed but not for more than 6 hours

Precautions Required for Blood Components Preparation Area

The precautions for blood components preparation are as follow:
Selection of area, maintain sterility, avoid pollution hazard and other precautions are very important for quality product. Some instructions are given below.
- The premises used for processing of blood components should be kept in a sterile, clean, and pollution-free area.
- As per the national guidelines components preparation area should be at least 50 square meters.
- Room should be fully air-conditioned and temperature to be maintained at 20–24°C.
- Component preparation should always be in a closed system to maintain sterility and avoid contaminations.
- One changing room should be there for sterile precaution.
- Before entering in the preparation area change shoe and wear disposable gloves, gown, cap, musk, etc.

Equipments and materials required for components preparation

1. Refrigerated centrifuge (See Figs 7.1A and B) .
2. Refrigerator for packed cell storage (See Fig. 15.1).
3. Deep freeze –40°C to – 80°C (See Fig. 8.4).
4. Platelet agitator incubator (See Figs 8.5A and B).
5. Electronic tube sealer (See Fig. 7.4).
6. Horizontal laminar airflow bench (See Fig. 7.2).
7. Electronic or manual plasma expresser (See Fig. 8.2A).
8. Weighing balance with double pan or electronic weighing machine (Figs 5.3A and B).
9. Weighing scale (Fig. 5.6).
10. Plasma thawing bath (See Fig. 7.3).
11. Cryobath for preparation of cryoprecipitate.
12. Biomedical waste disposal buckets with proper color codes.

Methodology of Blood Components Preparation 29

13. Plastic bar stick, clips, rubber band, etc. (See Figs 6.1A and B).
14. Sterile connecting device.
15. Blood group labels and components labels, etc.

*Hot air oven, autoclave machine, incubator, tap water, basin, ceiling fan, etc. should not be placed in a component processing area.

Outlet drainage is not allowed.

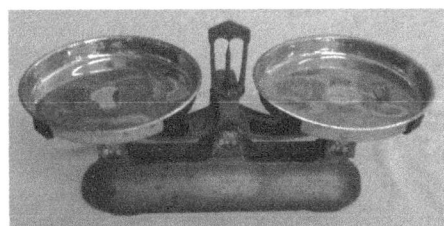

Figure 5.3A: Weighing balance with double pan

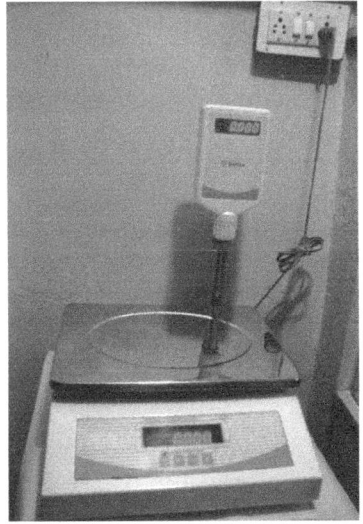

Figure 5.3B: Electronic weighing machine

Precautions Required for Blood Components Preparation

- For blood components preparation should maintain accurate collection volume of blood according to anticoagulants supply in the bag. It should be strictly followed for quality product (Fig. 5.4).
- For blood components preparation after collection of blood, keep at room temperature (20°C–24°C) till processed but not for more than 6 hours.
- Selection of time is very important for blood components preparation that is not more than 6 hours from collection of blood.
- For blood components preparation during collection, blood should be mixed properly with respective anticoagulants by automated shaker or gently shake by hand.
- According to the components to be prepared from the blood unit, donor selection, health and weight of the donor and selection of the bag is very important.
- Quality of the container and anticoagulant preservative solution.
- Technique of phlebotomy.
- Maintain storage temperature.
- For optimum quality component preparation whole blood required is 450 mL because optimum platelets yields and other coagulation factors yields are more available there (Fig. 5.4).
- Components room should be maintained at 20–24°C temperatures.
- Before collection of blood clean donor's vein with betadine solution and isopropyl alcohol to remove bacteria as much as possible (Fig. 5.1).
- During collection donor cuff pressure may be maintained at 70 mmHg for smooth blood flow.

Methodology of Blood Components Preparation **31**

- Components preparation is always done under laminar airflow bench with sterile condition, because bacterial contamination must be avoided (See Fig. 7.2).
- Before and after preparation of component, clean the laminar airflow bench.

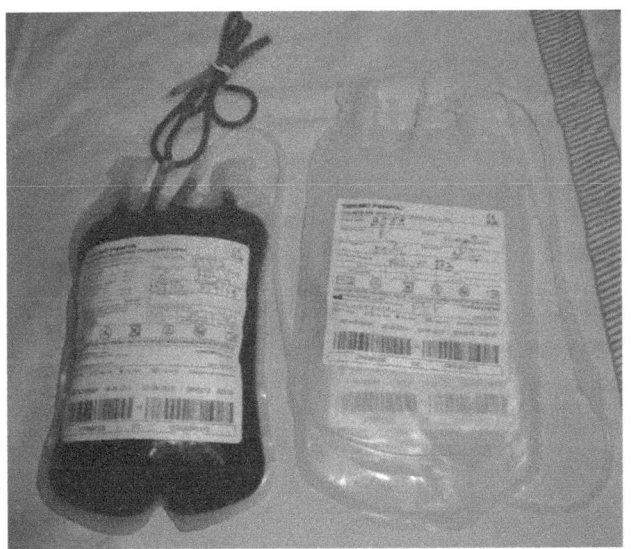

Figure 5.4: Whole blood (450 mL) in quadruple bags

Common Things to be Done Before Preparation of Blood Components

- A 450 mL triple bags or quadruple bags contain 63 mL of CPD preservatives (extra 100 mL SAGM-2) and a 350 mL single bag and double bags contains 49 mL of CPDA preservatives.
- Platelets concentrate should be separated from whole blood within 6–8 hours of collection (preferably 6 hours). At that time it should be kept at room tem-

perature (20–24°C). After preparation of platelets bag it should kept at room temperature for 1 hour and after that kept at 22–24°C platelet agitator incubator (See Figs 8.5A and B).

- Fresh frozen plasma component preparation, plasma should be separated from the whole blood not later than 6–8 hours of collection (preferably 6 hours). At the same time SAGM-2 preservative blood can be stored at 2–6°C temperature (blood bank refrigerator), and plasma bag should be storage at –80°C or lower for 24 hours. After solidifying transfer to –30°C chest deep freeze for one year.
- Cryoprecipitate component preparation should prepare from FFP component bag and FFP bag should be storage (rapidly freezing, blast freeze) at –80°C for 48 hours or below –80°C for 72 hours. Cryoprecipitate component is more available at –80°C blast freeze (See Fig. 8.4).
- After collection of blood, put knot in collection tube nearest to blood bag (downwards needle) and then seal into several segments by sealer machine.
- Remove adhered blood from the upper tubes of the bag by gently tapping.
- Collection tube should be rolled and clumped by rubber band (Fig. 5.4).
- According to preparation of respective component check and ensure that the donor number and other records in the mother bag and satellite bags are the same. The records which are written in the mother bag, also be mentioned in the satellite bags and logbook register.
- Keep blood bag gently in inner side of the bucket (surface of plain narrow area). Put satellite bags and collection tube in inner side of the bucket carefully

(surface of joint bucket's wide handle area). Because clips (locks) of handle can damage blood bag during centrifugation (Fig. 5.5A).
- Stroke gently by light hammering on top of the bag (glass sealer and upper tube). During this time RBC comes down and after centrifugation red cell contamination will not be there.
- If you collect blood and prepare respective component immediately then before centrifugation keep blood bag inside the bucket for minimum half an hour at room temperature. During this time RBC will be settled and production will be good.
- Before balancing the blood bag buckets, check weighing machine and place weighing needle at proper center of the machine (Fig. 5.5B).
- Balance the blood bags with buckets; weight of the opposite bucket should be equal.
- Accurate balance is done by plastic stick bar, plastic rod and final adjustment by pieces of soft plastic (See Fig. 6.1B).
- Remove blood group label and don't use plastic packet during keeping the bag inside the bucket and place the blood bag bucket inside the refrigerated centrifuge diagonally (opposite).
- If need to prepare only two bags component products then two pair of buckets should be used and blood bag bucket always be placed inside the center of centrifuge and empty bucket also be placed inside centrifugation wall (both blood bag facing same direction at center of centrifuge) (See Fig. 8.1).
- Before running refrigerated centrifuge check all parameters according to respective component programed and leave in running condition for half an hour. Dur-

ing this time compressor will start and help to reach required temperature.

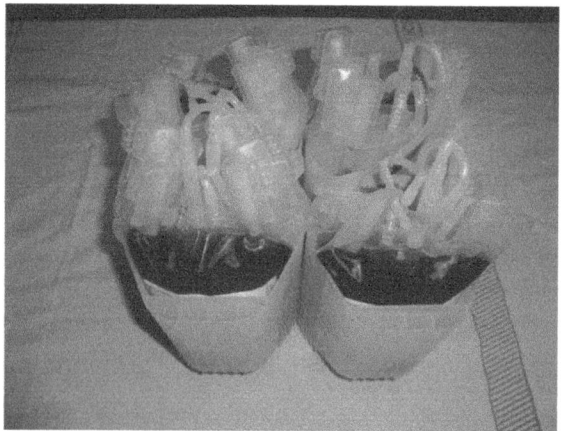

Figure 5.5A: Blood bags in buckets

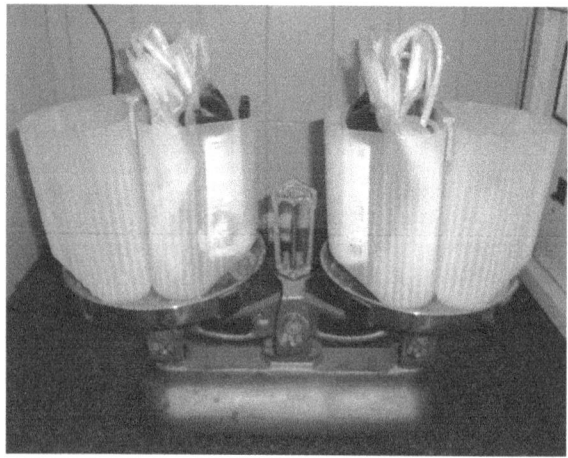

Figure 5.5B: Weighing balance with blood bags buckets

Common Things to be Done During Preparation of Blood Components

- During preparation of components horizontal laminar airflow bench should start before the work (See Fig. 7.2).
- Laminar bench, plasma expresser, weighing machine (for component product) and tubing sealer must be cleaned and in sterile condition.
- Plasma expresser, weighing balance (for component product), tubing sealer, plastic clips, marker, all materials are available inside the laminar bench during component preparation (Fig. 5.6. See Figs 6.1B, 7.4 and 8.2A).
- Do not use plastic clips during centrifugation; blood bag can be damaged or ruptured (See Fig. 6.1B).
- Take out respective component product with buckets from refrigerated centrifuge very carefully otherwise plasma will be mixed with RBC.
- Take out product bag from buckets very carefully; hold upper seal of the mother bag by thumb and index finger very tightly. Then turn up without disturbance and place on plasma expresser.
- Before breaking glass sealer of mother bag, check all records like blood group, blood bank number, unit number or product number name of component, date of collection and expiry of the collection of satellite bag and also check leakage of bag.
- Before breaking glass sealer of mother bag, if blood is visible on the top of the mother bag (inside glass seal and upper tube) leave the blood bag for few minutes on the plasma expresser to settle down RBC automatically.
- During preparation of product if hemolysis is visible discard plasma bag.
- During preparation of product if hyperactive color is visible (pale yellow) and bilirubin test result shows more than 1.2 mg%, plasma product is discarded.

- After separating respective component seal the tube by electric sealer two or three respective distance (See Fig. 7.4).
- During preparation of respective component after completing the collection of plasma in respective satellite bag, air must be released to mother bag or extra empty satellite bag.
- After completing preparation paste blood group label on mother bag and respective components label on component bags and keep it according to temperature.
- During preparation of component rubber band is used because in some manufacturing company, connecting tubes of satellite bags do not have any glass seal.

FFP component for pediatric patient

- During preparation of FFP component keep one satellite bag with FFP bag (and mark as transfer bag for pediatric patient). This satellite bag is used for pediatric patients according to needs of released volume of component measured by weighing scale (Fig. 5.6).

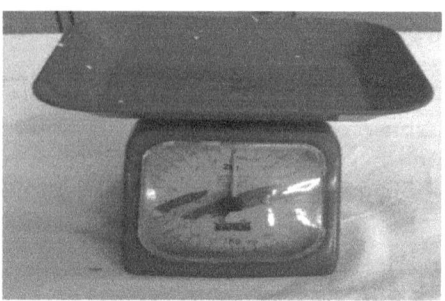

Figure 5.6: Weighing scale

Basic Informations for Blood Components Product

Chapter 6

Instruction Followed for Blood Components Preparation

- **Single donor for plateletpheresis**:
1. Platelet count should be determined before plateletpheresis and should be more than 1.5 lakhs.
2. Persons who have ingested aspirin or similar antiplatelet drugs in the last 72 hours are not suitable for plateletpheresis.

- **Important suggestion for platelets preparation from whole blood collection**:
1. Platelets concentrate preparation is done in triple bags system. Because among triple bags special satellite bag is made for platelets preparation.
2. If quadruple bags is used for platelets concentrate preparation, buffy-coat method is best for this preparation because platelets are more available in this method (See Fig. 5.4).
3. For leuko-depleted packed cells preparation quadruple bags are useful. Because extra satellite bags are made, and 100 mL SAGM-2 preservative extra are included there. Special satellite bag also be made for PLTC component preparation (See Fig. 5.4).
4. For PLTC component preparation refrigerated centrifuge should prerun at (22°C), 4,000 RPM, ACCL 9,

and DECL 6 for 10 minutes. During this time required temperature comes at (22°C). (RPM, TIME, ACCL and DECL can be changed according to needs because these parameters may differ from centrifuge to centrifuge) (See Figs 7.1A and B).
5. For platelet concentrate preparation selection of programs like RPM, TIME, ACCL and DECL depend on the use of bags. Select RPM, TIME, ACCL and DECL by experience and observation on good quality PLTC preparation. And also follow manufacturer's instruction (See Table 7.1).
6. During preparation of PLTC 2nd spin centrifugation, keep buffy-coat bag or PRP bag always inside the buckets in vertical position and packing should be done in buckets with thermocol. Because volume of buckets is larger but volume of above product in bags is very less amount.
7. Leuko-depleted packed cell can prepare by 'hard spin', i.e. 4,000 RPM, ACCL 8, and DECL 5 for 10 minutes or 3,500 RPM, ACCL 9, and DECL 6 for 15 minutes at 5°C. During separation of plasma for FFP/CRYO component it can easily be removed from RBC, and using this process technically one can try his best to reduce leukocytes in more percentage (See Figs 8.6A to F), (RPM, TIME, ACCL and DECL can be changed according to needs because these parameters may differ from centrifuge to centrifuge).

Cryoprecipitate component preparation from FFP bag

- After separation of cryopoor plasma by centrifugation remaining plasma with 15–20 mL white flakes (cryoprecipitate) should store again at –80°C for 1 year

and after thawing at 4°C temperature it can be used (See Fig. 8.4).
- For cryoprecipitate preparation, refrigerated centrifuge and cryowater bath instruments are more useful than hanging method procedure. Stable factors and unstable factors are more available in refrigerated centrifuge method. Because hanging method preparation takes more time (6–8 hours). In this time available factors are reduced.
- Cryopoor plasma (CPP) can be released for burn cases and hypoalbuminemia cases because albumin and globulin are available in CPP component. Approx 150 to 160 mL volume is available there.
- For FFP/cryoprecipitate/packed cell/saline washed RBCs refrigerated centrifuge should run for 30 minutes, i.e. 1,500 RPM, ACCL 9, and DECL 5 at 5°C for precooling. During this time required temperature reaches at 5°C, (RPM, TIME, ACCL and DECL can be changed according to needs because these parameters may differ from centrifuge to centrifuge).
- Platelet-poor plasma can be used as FFP. Except platelets all other coagulation factors are available in this preparation. Approx 180–200 mL volume is available there.
- In preparation of 350 mL packed cell bag if 50–60 mL plasma is available and in 450 ml of bag 70–80 mL plasma is available then the lifespan of RBC's do not change.
- FFP and cryoprecipitate component can be used upto 5 years if it is preserved and maintained in accurate temperature at –80°C (See Fig. 8.4).
- Always keep packed cells blood in horizontal position and also keep whole blood in vertical position (blood bank refrigerator) at 2°C–6°C temperature (See Fig. 15.1).

- Follow instructions for use of quadruple bags during centrifuge of 2nd spin. Keep mother bag and satellite bags inside the bucket gently. Keep plasma bag and extra preservative bag inside the other attached bucket. Same thing should be done in opposite balancing bucket because the above four bags will not be kept together inside a single bucket. It depends on size and capacity of buckets and packing should be done in buckets with thermocol because plasma bag and mother bag will be folded and settled at the bottom and there may be chance of mixing.
- For best product of component preparation quality of bag selection is very important, specially platelets concentrate preparation should be used in standard bags.
- In plasma available stable coagulation factors are fibrinogen, (FVII, FX, FXI, FXIII, etc.) and unstable (labile) factors are FV and FVIII.
- Various makes and models of refrigerated centrifuge are available with regards to capacity, rotor size, radius, etc. different. So programs like RPM, TIME, ACCL and DECL, vary and can be changed according to needs as per manufacturer's instruction and are documented in the manuals (See Table 7.1).
- Selection of bags like double bag, triple bag, and quadruple bag is used for preparation of respective component like FFP, cryoprecipitate, and PLTC, selection of suitable programe, RPM, TIME, ACCL and DECL. These can be changed according to guidance of manufacturer's instruction (See Table 7.1).
- For blood components preparation mainly two spins are used, i.e. 'light spin and hard spin'. For PLTC preparation (PRP method) 'light spin and hard spin'

are used (by buffy-coat method 'hard spin and light spin' are used). And for packed blood cell/leuko-depleted packed blood cell, FFP, and cryoprecipitate components only 'hard spin' is used. Various makes and models of refrigerated centrifuge are available with regards to capacity, rotor size, radius, etc. different. So programs like RPM, TIME, ACCL and DECL vary and can be changed according to needs as per manufacturer's instruction and are documented in the manuals (See Table 7.1).

Materials Required for Blood Components Product

- Double bags /triple bags and quadruple bags (See Fig. 5.4)
- Saline (0.85%)
- Transfusion set
- Transfer bag
- Bucket (See Fig. 6.1A)
- Scissors
- Pliers
- Forceps
- Clips (See Fig. 6.1B)
- Rubber band
- Marker
- Plastic bar stick/rod stick and soft plastic pieces (See Fig. 6.1B)
- Stripper (used to check platelet sampling quality)
- Gloves, cotton, and spirit.

> During preparation of product if hemolysis is visible discard plasma bag

Instrument materials required

- Blood bank refrigerator (See Fig. 15.1)
- Refrigerated centrifuge (See Figs 7.1A and B)
- Horizontal laminar airflow bench (See Fig. 7.2)

- Deep freeze –40°C to –80°C (See Fig. 8.4)
- Chest deep freeze –30°C to –40°C (See Figs 8.3A to C).
- Electronic or manual plasma expresser (See Fig. 8.2A).

> During preparation of product if hyperactive color is visible (pale yellow) and bilirubin test result shows >1.2 mg%, plasma product should be discarded.

- Weighing balance with double pan or electronic weighing machine (See Figs 5.3A and B).
- Electronic tube sealer (See Fig. 7.4).
- Platelet agitator incubator (See Figs 8.5A and B).

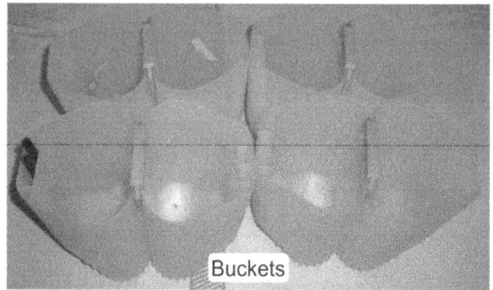

Figure 6.1A: Buckets

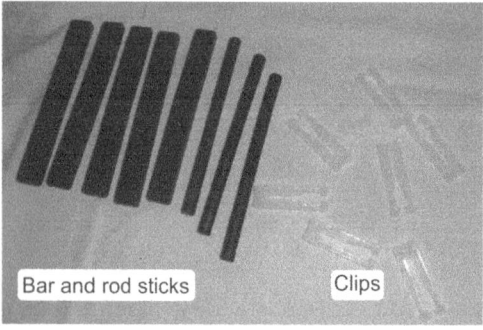

Figure 6.1B: Bar, rod sticks, and clips

- Refrigerated circulating plasma/cryowater bath, 4°C–37°C (See Fig. 7.3)
- Weighing scale (See Fig. 5.6)
- Saline stand
- P^H meter
- Blood group labels and component labels
- Biomedical waste bucket.

Safe Handling of Equipments

Chapter 7

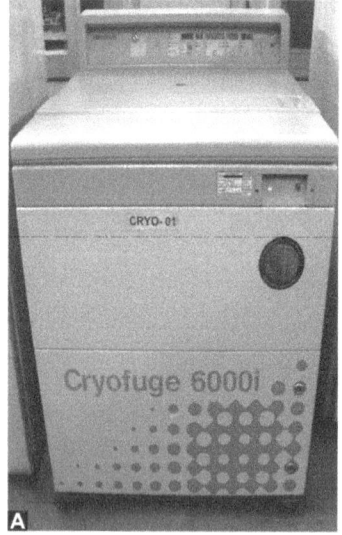
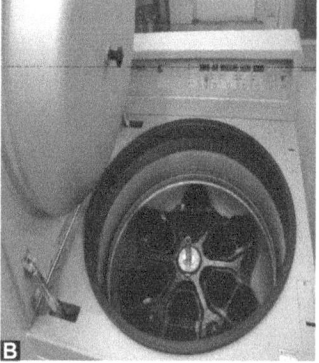

Figures 7.1A and B: Cryofuge 6000i refrigerated centrifuge

> Refrigerated centrifuge machine should be calibrated for every three months of interval

Refrigerated Centrifuge (Cryofuge 6000i)

Refrigerated centrifuge is an instrument which helps to separate components by different centrifugal force and different time. Radius and rotor of centrifuge are maintained by manufacturer, but RCF (relative centrifugal force), RPM, and TIME can be changed according to different products. If RPM is put in programing, RCF can be calculated automatically and if RCF is put in programing, RPM can be calculated automatically.

☐ **Calculation of following formula**:

$$RCF = \left(\frac{RPM}{1,000}\right) \times r \times 1.18 \Rightarrow RPM = \sqrt{\frac{RCF}{r \times 1.118}} \times 1,000$$

RCF = relative centrifugal force
RPM = rotational speed (revolutions per minute)
r = centrifugal radius in mm = distance from the center of the turning axis to the bottom of the centrifuge.

Programing of Cryofuge 6000i

Key switch function of cryofuge 6000i:
- Key mode A, B, C can be changed by key.
- Position 'A' key: Unlimited use of all sets possibilities. The user can alternate or use main programs and also save the program in program memory.
- Position 'B' key: The program memory is secured against alternations. The user can use but not alternate all programs. Only program number can be changed.
- Position 'C' key: The user cannot change program number and program memory. All set parameters are blocked, yet the current centrifugation program can be driven as often as needed with the control keys (start, stop, and open lid).

- Switch on the cryofuge refrigerator centrifuge and current will pass throughout the entire system and after few minutes compressor will start.
- In monitor (programed menu) speed 300 with blink, time hld is displayed.
- In this instrument 1–32 programed can be done.
- According to needs select ← (leftcresar) and → (rightcresar), ↑ (upcresar) and ↓ (downcresar) for programing.
- Radius and rotor of the centrifuge is already maintained by manufacturer.
- Select speed/ACCL/DECL/TIME/TEMPERATURE according to needs of programe and press store mode and button of execute. Then it is saved and program should check in memory buttom.
- If program is selected temporarily, then RPM/TIME/TEMPERATURE can change and press execute mode, but do not press store mode.
- If E-23 is displayed on the monitor stop cryofuge centrifuge immediately and start after 5–10 minutes interval.
- Various makes and models of refrigerated centrifuge are available with regards to capacity, rotor size, radius, etc. So programs like RPM, TIME, ACCL, and DECL vary and can be changed according to needs as per manufacturer's instruction and are documented in the manuals (Table 7.1).

Handling of Cryofuge Centrifuge 6000i and Other Models of Refrigerated Centrifuge

- Start the refrigerated centrifuge half an hour before the work according to program. During this time it will get the required temperature (Figs 7.1A and B).
- Before keeping blood bag buckets inside the refrigerated

centrifuge both balance and weight of the blood bags with buckets should be equal (See Fig. 5.5B).
- Place blood bag, satellite bags and tubing of the blood bag inside the bucket very carefully.
- Place pair of buckets with blood bag inside the cups in opposite direction (See Fig. 8.1).
- Before keeping blood bags and satellite bags inside bucket check all records like blood group/blood bank number/product number or unit number, etc. and mention the same on satellite bags according to product.
- Do not use plastic clips and plastic packet during centrifugation of bags because clips can damage the bags. Remove blood group label from mother bag before centrifugation (See Fig. 6.1B).
- Correct speed of centrifugation and time must be maintained as they are the most critical factors in component preparation.
- Observe for any abnormal vibration till the required speed is attained, if there is any, stop the refrigerated centrifuge and check the weight of opposite cups with component bags.
- If processor is sensed and any abnormal displayed on monitor like check lid, imbalance, system check, program error, and overtemperature, then it will stop automatically.
- In case of two bags preparation place both the bags in two buckets separately. Place blood bags with bucket inside the center of centrifuge in opposite direction (both blood bags face center of centrifuge) and keep empty bucket on the wall of the centrifuge.
- Thoroughly clean the bucket before keeping blood bag inside it.

- Select appropriate program depending upon the component to be prepared.
- Never start the refrigerated centrifuge when all of the carrying buckets are not inserted.
- After complete work of centrifuge clean by spirit cotton and dry it.
- After complete work of centrifuge close the lid and switch off the machine and main power.

> Do not use plastic clips during centrifugation; blood bag can be damaged or ruptured

> Various makes and models of refrigerated centrifuge are available with regards to capacity, rotor size, radius, etc. So programs like RPM, TIME, ACCL and DECL vary and can be changed according to needs as per manufacturer's instruction and are documented in the manuals.

Check Calibration of Cryofuge Centrifuge 6000i and Other Models of Refrigerated Centrifuge

☐ **Temperature**

1. Refrigerated centrifuge machine run for calibration of platelets preparation at 4000 RPM, ACCL 9, and DECL 6 for 10 minutes according to program number. During this time it gets the required temperature at 22°C. Stop the centrifuge machine, take glycerol in screw cap plastic container and keep container inside the centrifuge cup or bucket, close the lid and wait for 20–30 minutes. During this time temperature of inside centrifuge is shifted in glycerol container. Then insert a digital thermometer through a small hole of the cap of glycerol container and check the temperature of calibration at 22°C.

2. Refrigerated centrifuge machine run for calibration of FFP and cryoprecipitate component preparation at 4000 RPM, ACCL 9, and DECL 7 for 10 minutes at 4°C and check the temperature of calibration same as platelet calibration.

RPM, TIME, ACCL and DECL can be changed according to needs because these parameters may differ from centrifuge to centrifuge.

- **RPM**: Put a reflected paper inside the refrigerated centrifuge on center of the rod. Run the centrifuge machine at 4000 RPM, ACCL 9, and DECL 6 for 10 minutes. Measure the RPM from outside the hole by a tachometer, and check the RPM result. But the tachometer should be calibrated.

  RPM, TIME, ACCL and DECL can be changed according to needs because these parameters may differ from centrifuge to centrifuge.
  - The principle of calibration is same for other models of refrigerate centrifuge. But programs like RPM, TIME, ACCL and DECL, vary and can be changed according to needs as per manufacturer's instruction and are documented in the manuals. And machine should be calibrated for every three months of interval.
  - Refrigerated centrifuge are calibrated to produce highest product yield in the shortest time at the lowest possible spin so as to cause the least trauma to each product and at the same time maintaining optimal temperature for component viability (Figs 7.1A and B).

Table 7.1: Cryofuge centrifuge 6000i program of different blood component product

- 450 mL Whole Blood in Triple Bags/Quadruple Bags Collection

Component	ACCL	DECL	Speed (RPM)	RCF	Rotor	Radius	Time	Temp
Precooling Prog.(1)For PC/FFP/Cryo and Saline Wash Red Cell	9	5	1,500	0747	7617	29.7	30 min	5°C
Prog.(2) FFP/PC/Cryo	8	5	4,000	5313	7617	29.7	10 min	5°C
Prog.(3) FFP/PC/Cryo	9	6	3,500	4068	7617	29.7	15 min	5°C
Pre-run Prog.(4) For PLTC	9 Or 9	6 6	4,000 1,800	5134 5134	6694 6694	28.7 28.7	10 min 30 min	22°C 22°C
Prog.(5) Triple Bags PLTC (1st spin)	8	4	2,470	2026	6680	29.7	07 min	22°C
Prog.(6) PLTC (2nd spin)	8	4	4,000	4947	6680	29.7	10 min	22°C
Prog.(7) Cryoprecipitate	9	7	4,000	5313	7617	29.7	10 min	4°C
Prog.(2) Saline Washed Red Blood Cell	8	5	4,000	5313	7617	29.7	10 min	5°C

- 350 mL Whole Blood in Double Bags Collection

Component	ACCL	DECL	Speed (RPM)	RCF	Rotor	Radius	Time	Temp
Precooling Prog. (1)	9	5	1,500	0747	7617	29.7	30 min	5°C
Prog.(2) PC/FFP Saline-washed RBC	8	5	4,000	5313	7617	29.7	10 min	5°C

- Platelet Concentrate Preparation by PRP Method in Quadruple Bags:

Component	ACCL	DECL	Speed (RPM)	RCF	Rotor	Radius	Time	Temp
Pre-Run Prog. (4) For PLTC	9 Or 9	6 6	4,000 1,800	5134 5134	6694 6694	28.7 28.7	10min 30min	22°C 22°C
Prog. (8) PLTC(1St Spin)	9	6	1,800	1040	6694	28.7	10min	22°C
Prog. (9) PLTC(2Nd Spin)	9	6	4,000	5134	6694	28.7	10min	22°C
PC/FFP/Cryo/Saline-washed RBC	Same procedure should be followed as mentioned as in previous triple bags preparation							

- Selection of bags like triple bag and quadruple bag is used for preparation of platelet concentrate, selection of suitable programme RPM, TIME, ACCL and DECL. These can be changed according to guidance of manufacturer's instruction (See Table 7.1).
- During starting the refrigerated centrifuge machine for PLTC component preparation if the temperature shows below 10°C, at that time open the lid and rotor cover for 15 to 20 minutes at room temperature. Then close the lid, rotor cover and start pre-Run as per instruction. Temperature reaches at 22°C (See Figs 7.1A and B).

- Platelet Concentrate Preparation by Buffy-coat Method in Quadruple Bags:

Component	ACCL	DECL	Speed (RPM)	RCF	Rotor	Radius	Time	Temp
Prog.(4) Pre-Run for PLTC	9 Or 9	6 6	4,000 1,800	5134 5134	6694 6694	28.7 28.7	10 min 30 min	22°C 22°C
Prog. (10) PLTC (1st Spin)	9	6	3,800	1040	6694	28.7	09 min	22°C
Prog. (11) PLTC (2nd Spin)	7	5	850	5134	6694	28.7	09 min	22°C

- Various makes and models of refrigerated centrifuge are available with regards to capacity, rotor size, radius etc. different. So programs like RPM, TIME ACCL and DECL vary and can be changed according to needs as per manufacturer's instruction and are documented in the manuals (Table 7.1).

> Quadruple bags are used for all types of components like packed cells / leuko-depleted packed cell / FFP/ platelets concentrate and Cryoprecipitate. It can be used for preparation of leuko-depleted packed cells. 100 mL SAGM-2 preservatives are extra available in this bag

> Quadruple bags and triple bags are used for various types of component preparations like leuko-depleted packed cell/packed cell, FFP, cryoprecipitate and platelets concentrate. But selection of component preparation is important according to demand and supply

Horizontal Laminar Airflow Bench (Fig. 7.2)

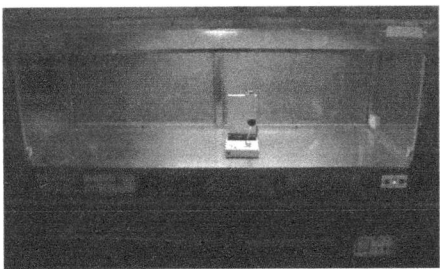

Figure 7.2: Laminar airflow bench

- Prepare respective components under laminar airflow bench with sterile condition. Ultraviolet ray kills the germs and blowers help to remove germs and sterile the working area.
- Start the laminar airflow bench one hour before the work.

54 Step by Step Technical Manual of Blood Components Preparation

- Before starting work clean laminar airflow bench regularly with betadine and isopropyl alcohol.
- After cleaning, switch on the cabinet tube light and UV light.
- Switch on the UV light upto 30 minutes which helps in sterilization of the chamber.
- When UV light is in running condition, close the front door.
- After starting UV light don't stand near laminar airflow bench because UV ray is harmful.
- After 30 minutes switch off the UV light and open the front door. Leave blowers running continuously till preparation of components.
- Now working area is ready for use. After finishing work again switch on the UV light and close front door upto 30 minutes.
- Switch off the UV light and open the front door.
- Then start blowers for 30 minutes.
- Switch off the blowers, clean the working area and switch off the cabinet light.
- After complete work clean the laminar bench with betadine and isopropyl alcohol.

Circulating Plasma/Cryowater Bath (Fig. 7.3)

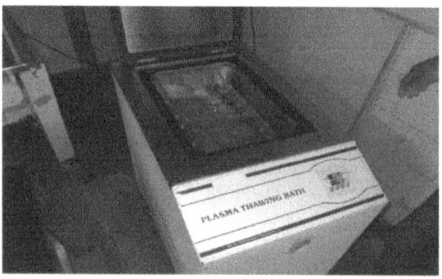

Figure 7.3: Cryowater bath

Handling of Circulating Plasma/Cryowater Bath

- Water bath has certain temperature; it helps to thaw respective components and temperature can change according to needs.
- Water should be changed when required.
- Temperature should be checked by thermometer.
- Start circulating cryowater bath for half an hour before taking out the respective components. During that time temperature will reach according to needs (4°C or 37°C).
- If thawed in a water bath, the entry ports must be protected so that water cannot contaminate the units.

Electronic Sealer (Fig. 7.4)

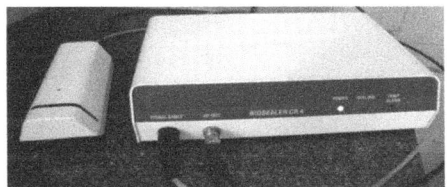

Figure 7.4: Electronic sealer

Operation of Electronic Sealer

- Electronic sealer is used for sealing blood bags and it helps to detach different component products.

Operation system

- It is kept on laminar chamber.
- Switch on the main point.
- After that switch on the sealer. When the power is on indicator is indicated green light.

- Tubing of the blood bag and component bags is placed gently on the slot and do not apply much pressure.
- Remove water pores tubing area by dry cotton.
- When the tubing is kept on the slot and indicate that sealing is completed, light is turned off automatically.
- Seal the tubing at more than two places.
- After the complete work turn the power off and clean the equipments.

Preparation of Blood Components—Procedures

Chapter 8

Blood Components Preparation (Flowchart 8.1)

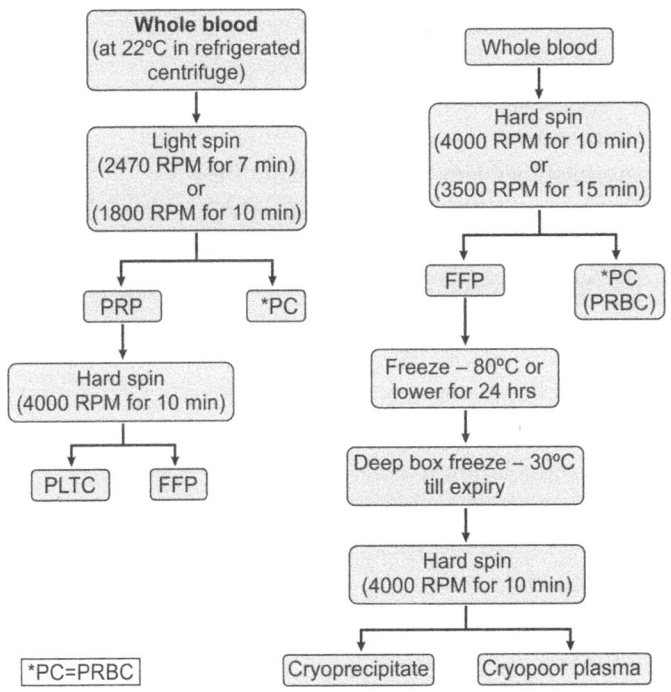

Flowchart 8.1: Blood components preparation

Packed Red Blood Cell (PRBC)/Fresh Frozen Plasma (FFP) by Double Bags Collection (Fig. 8.2B)

- **Principle**: A single unit of whole blood after 'heavy spin' should be separated of plasma and it should be frozen and preserved to have active coagulation factors at the appropriate temperature. Plasma must be prepared for freezing within 6–8 hours of phlebotomy (preferably 6 hours).

Materials Required

- Blood bank refrigerator (See Fig. 15.1).
- Double bags.
- Refrigerated centrifuge (cryofuge 6000i or other models) (See Figs 7.1A and B and Fig. 8.1).
- Deep freeze –80°C or lower (Fig. 8.4).
- Chest deep freeze –30°C to –40°C (Figs 8.3A to D).
- Plasma expresser (manual or electronic) (Fig. 8.2A).
- Weighing balance machine (double pan) or electronic weighing machine (See Figs 5.3A and B).
- Weighing balance scale (for product weight) (See Fig. 5.6).
- Horizontal laminar airflow bench (See Fig. 7.2).
- Electronic tube sealer (See Fig. 7.4).
- Bar sticks and rod sticks for balancing weight (See Figs 6.1A and B).
- Soft plastic pieces, plastic clips, marker, and rubber bands.

Preparation of Blood Components—Procedures

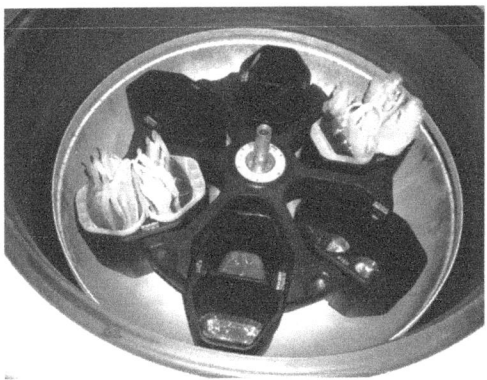

Figure 8.1: Cryofuge 6000i refrigerated centrifuge with blood bags bucket

1965- Cryoprecipitate was first used

To supply more safe blood to recipient in 1999 Nucleic acid amplification test (NAT) for HIV, Hepatitis B and Hepatitis C virus (HCV) infected blood from a donor in incubation period

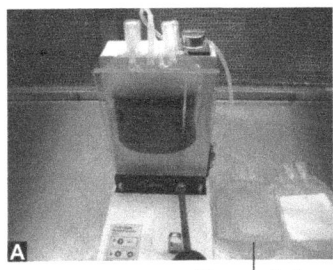
Plasma collection

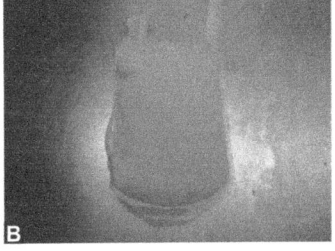

Figure 8.2A: Plasma expresser **Figure 8.2B**: Fresh frozen plasma (FFP)

FFP cannot be refrozen after thawing

14 mL of CPD/ CPDA-1 anticoagulant solutions is required for 100 mL of blood

- Scissors, light hammer, pliers, forceps, blood group labels and component labels.
- Gloves, cotton, and spirit.

> Keep blood bag gently inner side of the bucket (surface of plain narrow area). And put satellite bags and collection tube inner side of the bucket carefully (surface of joint bucket's wide handle area). Because clips (locks) of handle can damage blood bag during centrifugation

Procedure

- FFP is obtained from a single donor by donation.
- Collect appropriate volume of blood 350 mL in CPDA double bags system (49 mL preservative extra is also included there).
- Collect blood by a clean single vein puncture within 5–6 minutes.
- After collection of blood, store at room temperature (20–24°C) or 2–6°C till processed but not for more than 6 hours.
- After collection of blood put knot on the collection tube above the blood bag and then seal into several segments by sealer machine.
- Refrigerated centrifuge is put on for 30 minutes at 'light spin', i.e. 1,500 RPM, ACCL 9 and DECL 5 before starting the process. During this time required temperature reaches at 5°C. RPM, TIME, ACCL, and DECL can be changed according to needs because these parameters may differ from centrifuge to centrifuge (See Figs 7.1A and B).
- Check and ensure that the donor number and other records in the mother bag and satellite bag are the same.

- Collection tube should be rolled and clumped with rubber band and then insert under bucket with mother bag and satellite bag very carefully (without blood group label and plastic packet).
- Squeeze the tubing and stroke gently on glass sealer of the mother bag and remove adhered blood.
- Before taking weight of blood bag buckets check weight balance.
- Balance the blood bags with bucket on the monopan weight balance or electronic weighing machine.
- Weight of the opposite buckets should be equal (See Fig. 5.5B).
- In order to balance the blood bags in a bucket, use small plastic bar and plastic rod and adjust minutely by soft plastic pieces.
- Place the blood bag buckets of the refrigerated centrifuge diagonally in opposite positions.
- Close the lid of the refrigerated centrifuge and select the appropriate program on the centrifuge as per the need of the component prepared. Refer to the following chart for the application of the centrifugation speed, time, and temperature required to be given for the desired component.
- Start the refrigerated centrifuge at 'heavy spin', i.e. 3,500 RPM, ACCL 9, and DECL 6 for 15 minutes or 4,000 RPM, ACCL 8, and DECL 5 for 10 minutes at 5°C temperature. RPM, TIME, ACCL, and DECL can be changed according to needs because these parameters may differ from centrifuge to centrifuge (See Table 7.1).
- After centrifugation open the lid and take out the bag from the bucket and place on plasma expresser. Break the glass seal of the tubing connecting to the mother bag and collect maximum amount of plasma layer to flow out into the satellite bag and leave approx 50 to 60 mL of plasma in mother bag.

- Release air from plasma satellite bag by squeeze and transfer to mother bag and final volume of product is 160 to 180 mL (balance by weighing scale) (See Fig. 5.6).
- Seal the tubing by sealer and detach from mother bag and put knot on mother bag and again seal both the bags at minimum two respective distances.
- Paste blood group and respective component label in both the bags and check all the records.
- Packed cell is kept in the refrigerator at 2°C to 6°C in horizontal position and life of the blood is 35 days and component product (FFP) is kept in plastic packet and stored at –80°C or lower for 24 hours. After solidifying transfer to –30°C chest deep freeze for 1 year (Figs 8.3A and B).

> 1940 - Edwin Cohn – developed fractionation – plasma, albumin, protein

> An approved microwave thawing device can thaw FFP component at the temperature of 37°C (Sally V. Rudmann, page 247, 2nd edition)

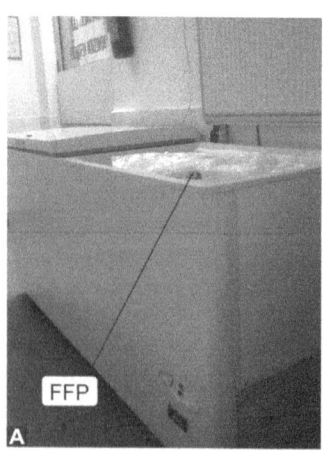
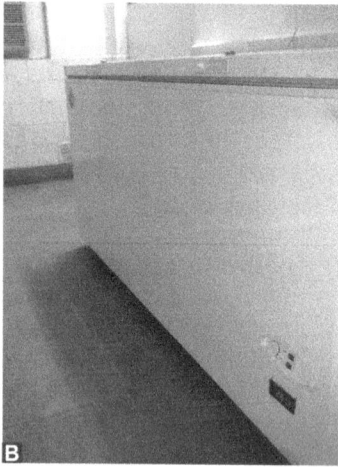

Figures 8.3A and B: –30°C chest deep freeze

> For best product of component preparation quality of bag selection is very important

> On March 27th, 1914, the first nondirect transfusion was performed by the Belgian doctor, Albert Hustin (was sodium citrate as an anticoagulant). After that on January 1st, 1916, the blood stored and cooled was transfused first time and practiced in 1917 when discovered the sodium citrate

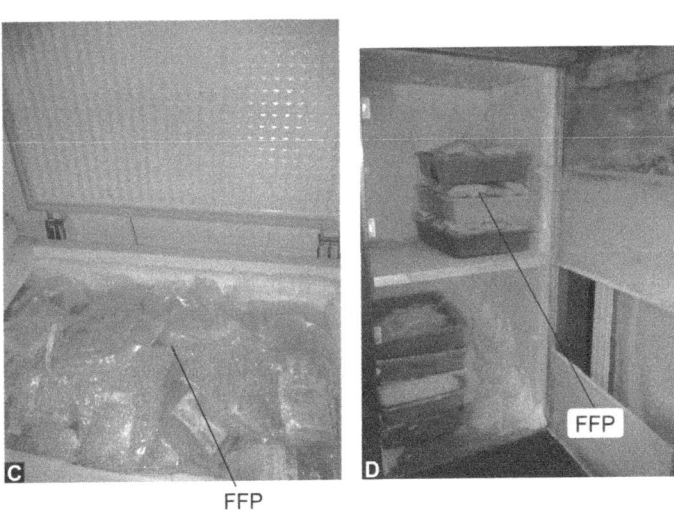

Figures 8.3C and D: C. –30°C chest deep freeze, and D.–30°C deep freeze

Leuko-depleted Packed Cell/Fresh Frozen Plasma by Triple Bags Collection

Procedure should be followed as same as previous mentioned steps in double bags FFP preparation. Few extra steps are included in triple bags preparation. Technically one can try his best to reduce buffy-coat with leukocytes from RBCs as much as possible (Figs 8.6A to D).

- Collect appropriate volume of blood 450 mL in CPDA–1 triple bags system (63 mL of preservative extra is also included there) and bind 2nd satellite bag tube with rubber band (if glass seal is not there) and mark as leukocytes collection.
- Balance the blood bags with bucket on the monopan weight balance or electronic weighing machine.
- Weight of the opposite buckets should be equal.
- Before placing blood bag buckets inside the refrigerated centrifuge, check temperature of refrigerated centrifuge at 5°C.
- Place the blood bag buckets of the refrigerated centrifuge diagonally in opposite positions.
- Start the refrigerated centrifuge at 'heavy spin' i.e. 3,500 RPM, ACCL 9, and DECL 6 for 15 minutes or 4,000 RPM, ACCL 8 and DECL 5 for 10 minutes at 5°C temperature. RPM, TIME, ACCL, and DECL can be changed according to needs because these parameters may differ from centrifuge to centrifuge (See Figs 7.1A and B).
- After centrifugation, collect maximum amount of plasma in 3rd satellite bag and clump immediately the tube by plastic clips.
- Remove rubber band or break the glass seal from 2nd satellite bag and collect buffy-coat with leukocytes and approx 15 to 20 mL RBCs as much as possible squeezing by finger very carefully at buffy-coat area from mother bag (Figs 8.6A to F; See Plate 3 for color Figure 8.6B and Plate 4 for color Figures 8.6C and F).
- Seal leukocytes bag by sealer and detach from mother bag and 3rd satellite bag and discard it (Flowchart 8.2).
- Hold 3rd plasma satellite bag and remove plastic clips from the bag and transfer approx 70–80 mL of plasma with air by squeezing process to mother bag and final volume of product will be approx 200–220 mL (Figs 8.2A and 8.6A). Detach plasma bag from mother bag and seal the tube by sealer.

- Remaining of this procedure will be followed the same as double bags FFP preparation.

Packed Red Blood Cell (PRBC)/Cryoprecipitate/ Cryopoor Plasma by Triple Bags Collection

Procedure should follow as same as previous mentioned steps of SOP double bags FFP preparation. Extra steps are included in triple bags preparation. Required materials are already mentioned on SOP of FFP.

Principle

- Coagulation factor VIII (antihemophilic factor—AHF), fibrinogen, von Willebrand factor, factor XIII, and fibronectin can concentrate from freshly collected plasma by cryoprecipitation. It is also prepared from fresh frozen plasma. Cryoprecipitation is accomplished by slow thawing at 2–6°C plasma that has been prepared for freezing within 6–8 hours of phlebotomy (preferably 6 hours).
- Collect appropriate volume of blood 450 mL in CPDA–1 triple bags.
- Bind 2nd satellite bag tube by rubber band (if glass seal is not there) and mark as CPP bag.
- Balance the blood bags with bucket on the monopan weight balance or electronic weighing machine.
- Weight the opposite buckets should be equal.
- Before placing blood bag buckets inside the refrigerated centrifuge, check temperature of refrigerated centrifuge at 4°C.
- Place the blood bag buckets of the refrigerated centrifuge diagonally in opposite positions.

Step I

- Start the refrigerated centrifuge at 'heavy spin', i.e. 3,500 RPM, ACCL 9, and DECL 6 for 15 minutes at 5°C or (4,000 RPM, ACCL 9, and DECL 7 for 10 minutes at 4°C temperature. This parameter is an ideal choice for cryopreparation). RPM, TIME, ACCL, and DECL can be changed according to needs because these parameters may differ from centrifuge to centrifuge (See Table 7.1).
- After centrifugation collect plasma in 3rd satellite bag and leave 70 to 80 mL of approx plasma in mother bag. Release air from 3rd satellite bag by squeezing process and transfer into mother bag, final volume is 200–220 mL (Figs 8.2A and 8.6A).
- Seal the tube at two points between the mother bag and Y connector and detach mother bag between the seal. Blood bag should be stored in horizontal position at 2–6°C temperature.

Cryoprecipitate Component Preparation

Step II

Plasma bag and attached satellite bag are kept in blast freeze at –80°C or lower for 1 year.

- Cryoprecipitate component is more available at –80°C blast freeze (Fig. 8.4).
- Take out solid plasma bag (FFP) from deep freeze and keep at room temperature for 5–10 minutes (during this time bag will be soft; if it is hard there will be possibility of leakage) and thaw at 4°C circulating cryo-water bath or at 4°C cold room/blood bank refrigerator.
- Solidify plasma bag is placed inside the circulating cryowater bath and hang attached satellite bag outside of the bath and during thawing component bags

should be kept inside plastic packet. It will thaw upto 30–45 minutes.
- Balance the thawed plasma bags with bucket on the monopan weight balance or electronic weighing machine (See Figs 5.3A and B).
- Weight of the opposite buckets should be equal. Packing should be done in buckets with thermocol because volume of buckets is larger.
- Before placing blood bag buckets inside the refrigerated centrifuge, check temperature of refrigerated centrifuge at 4°C.

Step III

- Keep thawed plasma in refrigerated centrifuge and start immediately at 'heavy spin', i.e. 4,000 RPM, ACCL 9, and DECL 7 for 10 minutes at 4°C temperature. RPM, TIME, ACCL and DECL can be changed according to needs because these parameters may differ from centrifuge to centrifuge (See Table 7.1).
- Place plasma bag on plasma expresser and remove rubber band or break the glass seal from 2nd satellite bag and transfer cryopoor plasma (CPP) in the bag. Leave 15–20 mL plasma with white flakes. Volume of CPP is available 150–160 mL.
- Cryopoor plasma is kept again at –80°C or lower for solidify and after 24 hours transfer to –30°C chest deep freeze. In this plasma albumin and globulin are available and it can release for burn and hypoalbuminemia cases.
- Cryoprecipitate if delayed issue then keep at 2–6°C blood bank refrigerator not more than 6 hours. White flakes will dissolve automatically at 25–30°C within 5–10 minutes or it should mix gently by hand and dissolve automatically within few minutes. After

dissolve it should issue immediately and should not keep again at 2–6°C temperature.

Cryoprecipitate component preparation by hanging method

For the preparation of cryoprecipitate from FFP, hang the FFP bags at 4°C cold room or disolved automatically blood bank refrigerator in upside down position with the empty satellite bag in a declamped position. The plasma starts draining down leaving a cryoprecipitate in the primary bag. 15–20 mL of plasma with white flakes mix leaves in primary bag (this leaves the cryoprecipitate adhering to the sides of the primary bag). The total draining time required is about 6–8 hours. After the plasma drains, heat seal the cryobag and store the cryopoor plasma at –80°C or lower and before issue, cryoprecipitate bag can be kept at 4°C temperature in blood bank refrigerator.

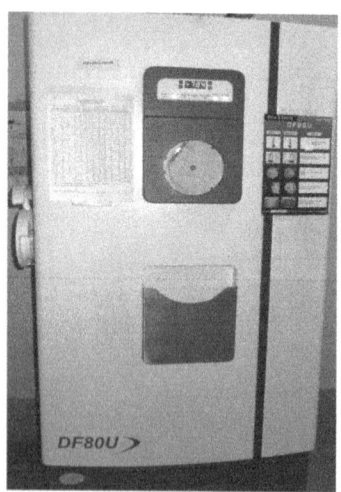

> The first blood bank establishing credit goes to Oswald Hope Robertson (was a medical researcher and US Army officer during World War I while he was serving at France

> Cryoprecipitate component is more available at –80°C blast freeze

Figure 8.4: –80°C blast deep freeze

Packed Red Blood Cell (PRBC)/Platelets Concentrate/ Platelets-poor Plasma/Fresh Frozen Plasma (PPP/FFP) by Random Donor in Triple Bags Collection

Principle

- Platelets are essential for the initial phase of hemostasis. Whole blood should undergo at 'light spin' centrifugation and from the platelet-rich plasma obtained platelet concentrate is prepared after 'heavy spin'. Platelets concentrate should be separated from whole blood within 6–8 hours of collection (preferably 6 hours).
- Before placing blood bag buckets in refrigerated centrifuge follow the procedure as in SOP of platelet preparation. Required temperature is 22°C and blood bag should be stored at room temperature. Remaining procedure is the same as previous mentioned component preparation. Extra steps are included there. Required materials are already mentioned on SOP of FFP (See Page no. 41 and 59).

Step I

- Collect 450 mL of whole blood in triple bags. Satellite bag is already marked for platelets collection. Bind 2nd satellite bag tubing by rubber band (if glass seal is not there) and mark platelets-poor plasma or FFP before placing inside buckets.
- After collection of whole blood it should separate within 6 hours of collection. During this time blood storage at room temperature (20–24°C, don't keep at 2–6°C blood bank refrigerator).
- Before placing blood bag buckets inside the refrigerated centrifuge, check temperature of refrigerated

centrifuge then start pre-run for 4,000 RPM, ACCL 9, and DECL 6 for 10 minutes at 22°C. During this time required temperature reaches at 22°C. RPM, ACCL, DECL, and TIME can be changed according to needs because these parameters may differ from centrifuge to centrifuge (See Figs 7.1A and B).

- Balance the blood bags with bucket on the monopan weight balance or electronic weighing machine. Weight the opposite buckets should be equal (See Figs 5.3A and B).
- Place the blood bag buckets of the refrigerated centrifuge diagonally in opposite positions.
- First run should at 'light centrifugation', i.e. 2,470 RPM, TIME, ACCL 8, and DECL 4 for 7 minutes or 1,800 RPM, ACCL 9, and DECL 6 for 10 minutes at 22°C. RPM, TIME, ACCL and DECL can be changed according to needs because these parameters may differ from centrifuge to centrifuge (See Table 7.1).
- Separate the available platelet-rich plasma (PRP) into a platelet collection satellite bag.
- Leave approx 70–80 mL of plasma in mother bag and release air from PRP bag and transfer into mother bag very carefully.
- After complete procedure seal mother bag and detach near Y junction from two satellite bags.
- Mix mother bag properly and keep blood bank refrigerator freeze at 2–6°C temperature; life of the blood is 35 days.

Step II

- PRP bag and attached satellite bag are placed again inside the bucket in vertical position without fold (packing should be done in buckets with thermocol) and balance these bags by weight machine.

- Start the refrigerated centrifuge at 'hard spin', i.e. 4,000 RPM, ACCL 8, and DECL 4 or ACCL 9, and DECL 6 for 10 minutes at 22°C temperature. RPM, TIME, ACCL and DECL can be changed according to needs because these parameters may differ from centrifuge to centrifuge. During centrifugation platelets will settle at the bottom of the bag because platelets are heavy.
- Place PRP bag on plasma expresser and remove rubber band or break the glass seal from 2nd satellite bag. Collect platelets-poor plasma in the bag.
- Approximate 50–60 mL of plasma is allowed to remain in platelets concentrate bag. After that follow the instructions of platelets preparation given in (See Page no. 74–76).
- Seal tubes on both the bags and detach from Y connector junction.
- Final volume of platelets-poor plasma (PPP) approx 180–200 mL should store at –80°C or lower for 24 hours. After that transfer plasma bag into chest deep freeze at –30°C till expiry and it can use as FFP.

> After starting UV light don't stand near laminar airflow bench or don't keep open the lid because UV ray is harmful

Packed Red Blood Cell (PRBC) (Leuko-depleted)/Platelets Concentrate by (Buffy-coat Method)/FFP Preparation in Quadruple Bags

Before preparation of platelets concentrate instruction of steps should be followed like triple bags preparation of PLTC. Platelets concentrate should be separated from whole blood within 6–8 hours of collection (preferably 6 hours).

Step I

- Collect 450 mL of whole blood in quadruple bags.
- Mark in 2nd satellite bag for FFP collection and SAGM–2 preservative bag for PLTC collection, bind 3rd satellite bag tubing by rubber band (if glass seal is not there) and mark for buffy-coat plasma collection.
- Balance the blood bags with bucket on the monopan weight balance or electronic weighing machine. Weight the opposite buckets should be equal (See Figs 5.3A and B).
- Place the blood bag buckets of the refrigerated centrifuge diagonally in opposite positions (Fig. 8.1).
- Before placing blood bag buckets inside the refrigerated centrifuge, check temperature of refrigerated centrifuge at 22° C.
- Start the refrigerated centrifuge at 'hard spin', i.e. 3,800 RPM, ACCL 9, and DECL 6 for 9 minutes at 22°C. RPM, TIME, ACCL and DECL can be changed according to needs because these parameters may differ from centrifuge to centrifuge (See Table 7.1).
- Place the mother bag on plasma expresser and transfer the available plasma (FFP) into 2nd satellite bag. And leave approx 50–60 mL (or one inches plasma with buffy-coat) of plasma into mother bag and clump immediately FFP bag tubing connector by plastic clip.
- Remove rubber band or break the glass seal from 3rd satellite bag and transfer available plasma with buffy-coat from mother bag into 3rd satellite bag. Squeeze or press surface of the buffy-coat area by finger very carefully and transfer maximum amount of buffy-coat with 15 to 20 mL of RBCs. After collection clump immediately mother bag tubing connector by plastic clip (near Y connector).
- Hold FFP bag and remove clump from this bag and release air with little amount of plasma transfer into

buffy-coat plasma bag (3rd satellite bag). This plasma will help to clean RBCs and buffy-coat in between connected tubing area and clump buffy-coat plasma bag connected tubing by plastic clip. Seal FFP bag tubing connector by sealer and detach FFP bag from mother bag, 3rd satellite bag and extra preservative bag. Final volume of product is approx 200 mL, then storage at −80°C or lower for 24 hours. After that transfer to −30°C chest deep freeze till expiry.
- Remove clip from mother bag and transfer all extra preservative (SAGM-2) into mother bag. After mixing properly detach mother bag from 3rd satellite bag and empty preservative bag (SAGM-2). Then blood bag should store at 2–6°C temperature.
- After transfer extra preservative into mother bag bind empty SAGM–2 bag connector tubing by rubber band. During hanging both the bags (empty preservative and buffy-coat plasma bag) avoid chance of contamination because adhering preservative may drain through connector tube and mix with buffy-coat plasma bag.

Step II

- Hang 3rd satellite bag (buffy-coat plasma bag) and connected empty preservative bag upto 1–2 hours. Hang empty bag in upwards direction and buffy-coat plasma bag in a downward position. During this time RBCs and buffy-coat will settle at the bottom.
- Buffy-coat bag and connected empty preservative bag are placed again inside the bucket and balance these bags by weight machine.
- Keep buffy-coat bag always inside the buckets in vertical position (without fold) and packing should be done in buckets with thermocol because volume of buckets is larger but volume of buffy-coat with plasma in bag is very little in amount. During centrifugation buffy-coat

plasma bag will be folded and settled at the bottom and there may be chance of mixing or contamination.
- Start the refrigerated centrifuge at 'light spin', i.e. 850 RPM, ACCL 7, and DECL 5 for 9 minutes at 22°C. RPM, TIME, ACCL and DECL can be changed according to needs because these parameters may differ from centrifuge to centrifuge.
- After centrifugation takes out the bag from bucket very carefully.
- Place buffy-coat plasma bag on plasma expresser and remove rubber band from empty preservative bag and transfer platelets concentrate into this bag, seal PLTC connected tubing by sealer and detach from buffy-coat, RBCs bag.
- Buffy-coat, RBCs bag will be discarded. After preparation of platelets concentrate available volume is 50–60 mL and remaining instruction should be followed as same as triple bags PLTC preparation (instructions of platelets preparation is given below.

The above-mentioned method is the best method for PLTC preparation in quadruple bags because optimum platelets yields are available there.

Instruction follows after Preparation of Platelet Concentrate in Triple Bags and Quadruple Bags

- After preparation of PLTC do not keep immediately inside the platelet agitator incubator. After preparation of bag it should not be used a minimum of 1 hour because during this time platelets generally aggregate together at bottom of the bag, so it is necessary to put the pump on the bag's surface and rub gently few minutes for spreading platelets uniformly.

- Platelets are resuspended by gently mixing and kept at 22–24°C in a platelets incubator with agitator until issue. Keep single bag inside the agitator incubator. Don't overlap the bags.
- PLTC bags are always kept under agitator incubator in horizontal position and plain surface of the bag is placed in upwards direction because oxygen is supplied through pores (Figs 8.5A and B; See Plate 3 for color Figure 8.5B).
- Continuous agitation 70–72 stroke/minutes should be maintained throughout the storage period.
- Reddish tinge of the concentrate indicates red cell contamination.
- Platelets should be suspended in approximately 50–60 mL of plasma and stored at 22–24°C. The P^H must be 6 or higher at the end of permissible storage period in all the platelets concentrate unit.
- There should be no grossly visible platelets aggregates during the storage. Swirling phenomenon should be checked before issue.
- Self-life of platelets is 5 days from time of whole blood collection.

Important points

- For storage of platelet the process recommended as per AABB* standards is platelet agitator/incubators provides a conductive environment.
- Safe storage of platelet concentrates through continuous agitation and in controlled temperature.
- Ensures no platelet clumping and maximum validity of platelets by uniform agitation.

*American Association of Blood Banks, 15th ed. 2005.

- For improving safety the agitation motion monitoring system is used.
- With the help of a unique airflow system the digital temperature recorder control unit is coupled for maintaining the chamber uniformly at AABB recommended temperature of 22°C ± 2°C.
- For matched exact temperature and also ensuring error-free readings inside the bag, the digital sensor placed inside the solution-filled bottle.
- To avoid platelet and to ensure maximum validity, agitation must be at 60 ± 5 cycle per minute.
- The sliding steel trays must be of SS304 grade.
- For easy placement and removal of bags pause switches has been used, which provides the arrest agitator motion for 10 seconds.
- Used glass door for safety and better visibility of platelet bags.
- Magnetic gaskets is used for doors to ensure no air transactions.
- When the door is opened the internal fan switches off to avoid the cold air moving out.
- TRUC positioned on eyelevel for better visibility.
- Auto light on system for better visibility when door is opened.
- Stabilizer protects the incubator from high/low voltage for long-life.

Buffy-coat method for PLTC preparation in quadruple bags is best method because optimum platelets yields are available there

---

Platelet count from 450 mL whole blood should > 4.5 ×10^{10}/unit (it also depends on platelet count of the individual donor and area)

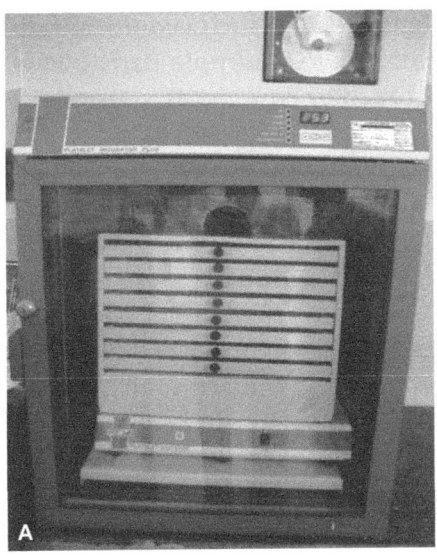

Safe storage of platelet concentrates by continuous agitation and controlled temperature

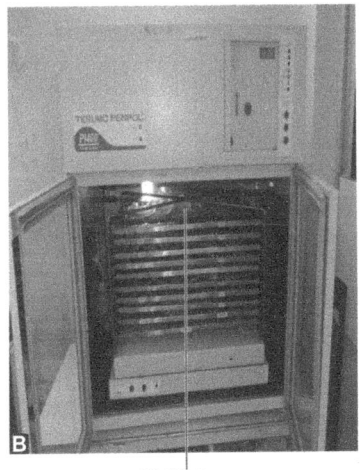

PLTC bags

In 1674, Antonie van Leeuwenhoek discovered the platelets

Figures 8.5A and B: Platelet agitator incubator

Leuko-depleted Packed Cell, FFP and Cryoprecipitate Components Preparation by Quadruple Bags (Flowchart 8.2; See Plate 2 for color Flowchart)

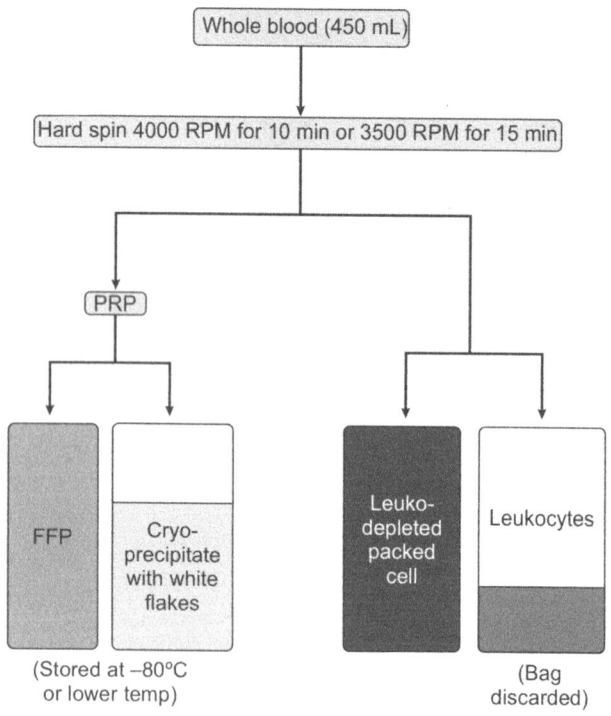

Flowchart 8.2: Blood components preparation by quadruple bags

RPM, TIME, ACCL and DECL can be changed according to needs because these parameters may differ from centrifuge to centrifuge.

For leuko-depleted packed cells preparation quadruple bags are very useful.

* Packed Red Blood Cell = PRBC

Preparation of leuko-depleted packed cells through pictures

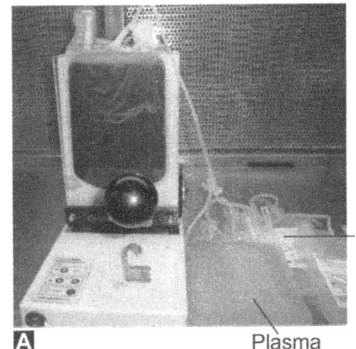

A — Leukocytes collection bag; Plasma

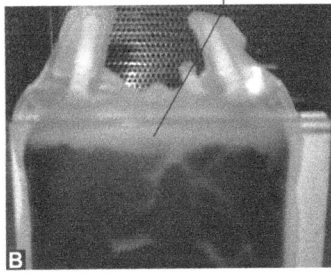

B — Buffy-coat with leukocytes

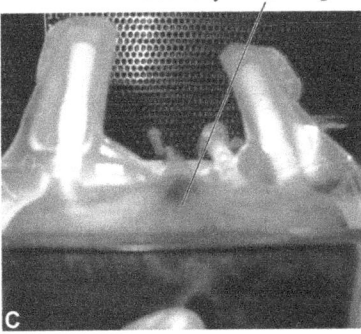

C — Leukocytes coming out

80 Step by Step Technical Manual of Blood Components Preparation

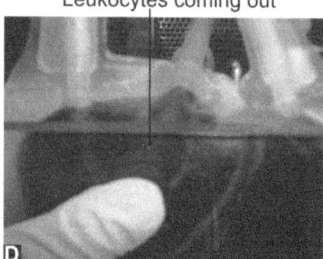

Leukocytes coming out

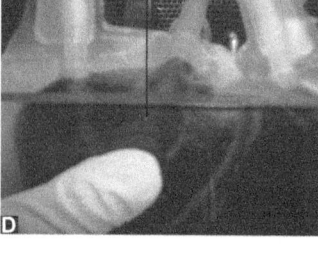

Leuko-depleted packed cells

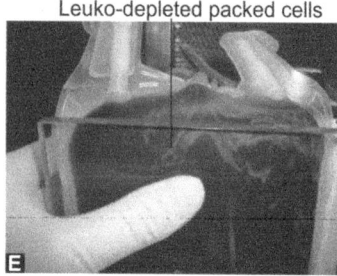

Leuko-depleted packed cells

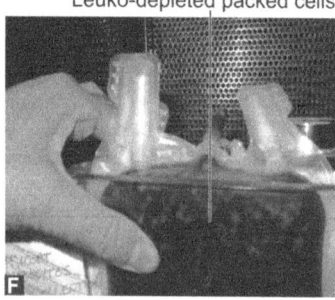

Figures 8.6A to F: A. Plasma; B. Buffy-coat with leukocytes; C and D. Leukocytes coming out; E and F. Leuko-depleted packed cells

*Preparation of leuko-depleted packed cells: Technically one can try his best to reduce buffy-coat with leukocytes from RBCs as much as possible.

Packed Red Blood Cell (Leuko-depleted), Fresh Frozen Plasma/Cryoprecipitate by Quadruple Bags (SAGM-2/ Adsol Preservative) (Flowchart 8.2)

Procedure should be followed like double bags preparation of FFP. Extra instruction and steps should be included there. Required materials are already mentioned on SOP of double bags FFP preparation.

- Collect 450 mL of whole blood in quadruple bags and bind rubber band in 2nd satellite bag (if glass seal is not there) and mark for leukocytes collection.
- Balance the blood bags with bucket on the monopan weight balance or electronic weighing machine. Weight the opposite buckets should be equal (See Fig. 5.5B).
- Before placing blood bag buckets inside the refrigerated centrifuge, check temperature of refrigerated centrifuge at 5°C.
- Place the blood bag buckets of the refrigerated centrifuge diagonally in opposite positions.
- Start the refrigerated centrifuge at 'heavy spin', i.e. 3,500 RPM, ACCL 9, and DECL 6 for 15 minutes or 4,000 RPM, ACCL 8, and DECL 5 for 10 minutes at 5°C temperature. RPM, TIME, ACCL, and DECL can be changed according to needs because these parameters may differ from centrifuge to centrifuge (See Figs 7.1A and B).
- Place mother bag on plasma expresser and collect maximum amount of plasma in 3rd satellite bag and mark as FFP component. After collection of plasma close FFP bag immediately the tubing connector by plastic clips.
- Remove rubber band or break the glass seal from 2nd satellite bag and collect buffy-coat with leukocytes and approx 15 to 20 mL RBCs as much as possible squeezing

by finger very carefully at buffy-coat area from mother bag (Figs 8.6A to D).
- Seal leukocytes bag by sealer and detach from mother bag and discard the bag.
- Remove plastic clips from FFP satellite bag and hold immediately FFP bag. Squeeze and transfer few mL of plasma with air to mother bag and final volume of FFP component is 220–250 mL.

> For various types of blood component preparation like FFP, PLTC and cryoprecipitate mainly two spins are used, i.e. "light spin and hard spin".

Cryoprecipitate component preparation

- After transfer of plasma with air, again clump tubing by plastic clips in FFP bag.
- Break the glass seal of the tubing connecting SAGM-2/ADSOL bag. And transfer all preservative into mother bag and mix gently.
- Detach mother bag from empty satellite bag and FFP bag. Blood bag should be stored at 2–6°C blood bank refrigerator and life of the blood is 42 days (used SAGM-2 or ADSOL preservative).
- FFP and attached empty satellite bag should be stored at –80°C blast freeze or lower (during storage empty bag should bind by plastic clips or rubber band).
- From FFP component, cryoprecipitate component can prepare and empty bag can use for collection of cryopoor plasma.
- For cryo component preparation always keep FFP bag at –80°C blast freeze. Cryo is more available in this freeze (Fig. 8.4).
- Remaining procedure of cryoprecipitate component preparation should be followed as same as previous-mentioned triple bags cryoprecipitate component.

- For FFP component preparation FFP bag should store at –80°C or lower for 24 hours and after that transfer to –30°C chest deep freeze for one year (Figs 8.3A and B).

> Prepared FFP component bag is used for pediatric patients and transfer amount of component to the attached empty satellite bag according to needs of released volume of FFP component measured by weighing scale

> For PLTC and cryoprecipitate component preparation packing should be done in buckets with thermocol because volume of buckets is larger. During centrifugation bag will be folded and settled at the bottom and there may be chance of mixing

Blood components preparation by quadruple bags (Flowchart 8.3)

Platelets poor plasma can use as FFP.

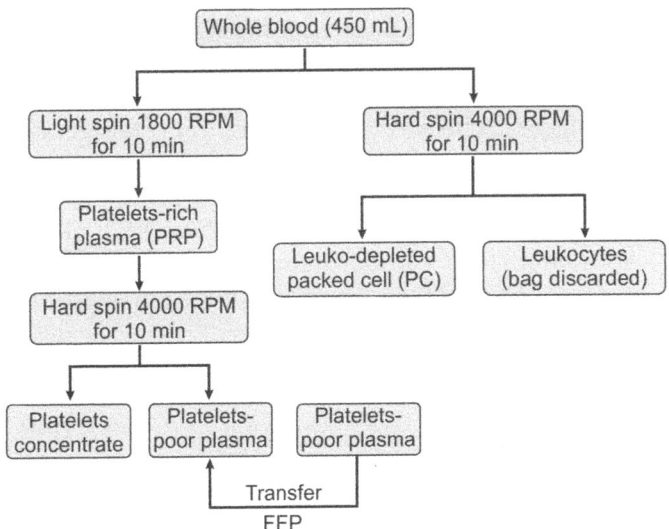

*Platelets poor plasma can use as FFP

Flowchart 8.3: Blood components preparation by quadruple bags

Packed Red Blood Cell (Leuko-depleted)/Platelets Concentrate by (PRP Method) and Platelet-poor Plasma (PPP/FFP) in Quadruple Bags (Flowchart 8.3)

Procedure and instruction of steps should be followed like triple bags preparation of platelets concentrate. Extra instruction of steps should be included there.

Step I

- Collect 450 mL whole blood in quadruple bags and bind rubber band in 2nd satellite bag (if glass seal is not there) and mark for leukocytes collection.
- Balance the blood bags with bucket on the monopan weight balance or electronic weighing machine. Weight the opposite buckets should be equal.
- Place the blood bag buckets of the refrigerated centrifuge diagonally in opposite positions.
- Before placing blood bag buckets inside the refrigerated centrifuge check temperature of refrigerated centrifuge, then start prerun, i.e. 4,000 RPM, ACCL 9, and DECL 6 for 10 minutes at 22°C. During this time required temperature reaches at 22°C. RPM, TIME, ACCL and DECL can be changed according to needs because these parameters may differ from centrifuge to centrifuge (See Figs 7.1A and B).
- Start the refrigerated centrifuge at 'light spin', i.e. 1,800 RPM, ACCL 9, and DECL 6 for 10 minutes or 2,470 RPM, ACCL 8 and DECL 4 for 7 minutes at 22°C. RPM, TIME, ACCL and DECL can be changed according to needs because these parameter may differ from centrifuge to centrifuge (See Figs 7.1A and B and Table 7.1).
- Separate the available platelets-rich plasma (PRP) into a platelets collection satellite bag. After collection

close immediately, bind tubing by rubber band and both mother and PRP bags.

Step II

- Mother bag, PRP bag, 2nd satellite bag, and extra preservative bag are placed again inside the bucket and should balance by weight machine.
- Keep mother bag and satellite bags inside the bucket gently. Keep plasma bag and extra preservative bag inside the attached other bucket. Same thing should be done in opposite balancing bucket because the above four bags will not be kept together inside a single bucket. It depends on size and capacity of buckets and packing should be done in buckets with thermocol because plasma bag and mother bag will be folded and settled at the bottom and there may be chance of mixing.
- Start the refrigerated centrifuge at 'hard spin', i.e. 4,000 RPM, ACCL 9, and DECL 6 for 10 minutes at 22°C temperature. During centrifugation platelets will settle at the bottom of the PRP bag. RPM, TIME, ACCL, and DECL can be changed according to needs because these parameters may differ from centrifuge to centrifuge (See Figs 7.1A and B and Table 7.1).
- Place the mother bag on plasma expresser; remove rubber band from mother and PRP bags. Collect remaining clear plasma (if available) into PRP bag and clump immediately PRP bag by plastic clips.
- Remove rubber band or break the glass seal from 2nd satellite bag and collect buffy-coat with leukocytes from mother bag as much as possible (Figs 8.6C and D).

- Detach buffy-coat, leukocytes bag by sealer and discard it.
- Break the glass seal of the tubing connecting SAGM-2/ADSOL bag and transfer all preservative into mother bag and clump empty bag by clips.
- Mix well and detach mother bag from empty preservative bag and PRP bag. Blood bag should store at 2–6°C temperature.

Step III

- Place PRP bag on plasma expresser and remove clips from PRP bag.
- Collect platelets-poor plasma in empty preservative bag. Leave 50–60 mL plasma with platelets in PRP bag.
- Detach both the bags by sealer. PRP bag is used for platelets concentrate. And platelets-poor plasma should store as FFP. Final volume of PPP is 180–200 mL.
- After preparation of PLTC, instruction should be followed as same as previous-mentioned triple bags platelet preparation (instruction is given on pages 74 and 75).

> For leuko-depleted packed cells preparation quadruple bags are usually used. Because extra satellite bags are made, and 100 mL SAGM–2 extra preservative are included there. Special satellite bag also be made for PLTC component preparation

Blood components preparation by quadruple bags (Flowchart 8.4)

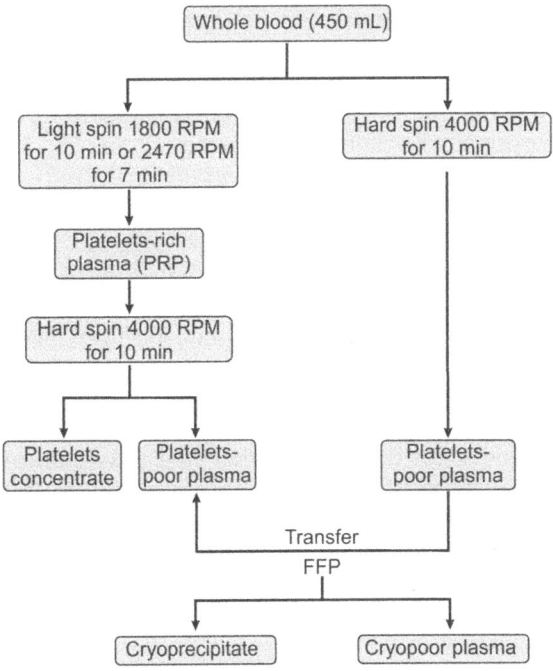

Flowchart 8.4: Blood components preparation by quadruple bags

Packed Red Blood Cell (PRBC)/Platelets Concentrate by (PRP Method)/Platelet-poor Plasma (PPP/FFP)/Cryoprecipitate or Required Amount of FFP for Pediatrics Patient in Quadruple Bags

Procedure and instruction should be followed as previousmentioned quadruple bags preparation. Remaining procedures are given on next page.

Step I

- Collect 450 mL of whole blood in quadruple bags and bind rubber band in 2nd satellite bag (if glass seal is not there) and mark FFP/cryoprecipitate or FFP for pediatric patients.
- Balance the blood bags with bucket on the monopan weight balance or electronic weighing machine. Weight the opposite buckets should be equal (See Fig. 5.5B).
- Before placing blood bag buckets inside the refrigerated centrifuge, check temperature of refrigerated centrifuge at 22°C.
- Place the blood bag buckets of the refrigerated centrifuge diagonally in opposite positions.
- Start the refrigerated centrifuge at 'light spin', i.e. 1,800 RPM, ACCL 9, and DECL 6 for 10 minutes or 2,470 RPM, ACCL 8, and DECL 4 for 7 minutes at 22°C temperature. RPM, TIME, ACCL and DECL can be changed according to needs because these parameters may differ from centrifuge to centrifuge (See Figs 7.1A and B and Table 7.1).
- Separate the available platelet-rich plasma (PRP) into 3rd satellite bag (marked PLTC as PRP bag).
- After collection of PRP in 3rd satellite bag close immediately, bind tubing by rubber band.
- Transfer extra preservative SAGM–2 into mother bag mix well and detach mother bag from remaining satellite bags.
- Blood bag should be stored at 2–6°C blood bank refrigerator.
- Bind tubing empty preservative bag by rubber band.

Step II

- 2nd satellite bag, PRP bag and empty preservative bag are placed again inside the bucket in vertical position

without fold. Packing should be done in buckets with thermocol because volume of buckets is larger and should balance by weight machine.
- Start the refrigerated centrifuge at 'hard spin', i.e. 4,000 RPM, ACCL 9, and DECL 6 for 10 minutes at 22°C temperature. During centrifugation platelets will settle at the bottom of the PRP bag. RPM, TIME, ACCL and DECL can be changed according to needs because these parameters may differ from centrifuge to centrifuge.
- Place PRP bag on plasma expresser and remove rubber band from PRP bag and break the glass seal or remove rubber band from 2nd satellite bag (FFP/Cryo or FFP for pediatrics).
- Collect platelets-poor plasma (PPP) in 2nd satellite bag. It can be use as FFP.
- Leave 50–60 mL plasma with platelets into PRP bag.
- Detach platelets concentrate bag from FFP and SAGM-2 empty bag.
- Mark on SAGM-2 empty satellite bag as transfer of FFP for pediatric patient or cryopoor plasma component collection bag.

Step III

- Keep both the attached bags (FFP bag and satellite transfer bag for pediatric patient) at –80°C Blast freeze for 24 hours. After that transfer to –30°C chest deep freeze till expiry. Volume of FFP is 200 to 220 mL (Figs 8.2A and 8.6A).
- If prepare cryoprecipitate component from FFP bag then keep both the attached bags (FFP and satellite bag) at –80°C blast freeze for 1 year (Fig. 8.4).
- Cryoprecipitate and platelets concentrate preparation instructions should be followed the same as previous mentioned procedure.

Step IV

- Prepared FFP component bag is used for pediatric patients and transfer amount of component to the attached empty satellite bag according to needs of released volume of FFP component measured by weighing scale (See Fig. 5.6).

Important information

1. Quadruple bags and triple bags are used for various types of component preparations like leuko-depleted packed cell/packed cell, FFP, cryoprecipitate and platelets concentrate. But selection of component preparation is important according to demand and supply.

Quadruple bags are also used as a transfer for pediatric patients' required amount of FFP.

Saline-washed Packed Red Blood Cell (PRBC) in Double Bags Preparation (450 mL/350 mL)

☐ **Function**: Washing of RBC blood bag with normal saline (sterile) for transfusion to thalassemia patient. Washed RBC can produced by automated cell washer or by centrifugation.

Material required

- Refrigerated centrifuge machine (See Fig. 15.1).
- Horizontal laminar airflow bench (See Fig. 7.2).
- Weighing machine (See Figs 5.3A and B).
- Stick bar/ rod bar/ soft plastic rubber pieces (See Figs 6.1A and B).
- Saline stand.

- Cold normal saline 0.85% (patient uses sterile N/S bottle).
- Transfusion sets.
- Transfer bag (double bags are used for 350 mL blood and for 450 mL blood triple or quadruple satellite bag are used) (See Fig. 5.4).
- Electronic tube sealer (See Fig. 7.4).
- Gloves, cotton, scissor, spirit, and forceps.

Principle

When we washed RBC, it removes all plasma, leukocytes and platelets from the original unit. It can be washed by using and automated cell washer or by centrifugation. The RBC is mixed with a large volume of physiologic saline. Then the mixture is centrifuged and the supernatant is removed. In this process about 99% of plasma protein and upto 20% RBC will be removed. It also removes 70% to 95% of the leukocytes depending on the methodology. When the washing process is completed, the RBC suspended in 0.85% normal saline. An addition of saline to blood bag and centrifuged, RBC is settled down, a layer of WBC is above RBC, that is called buffy-coat. Washing of RBC is indicated to eliminate the adverse anaphylactic reaction to plasma proteins mainly specially in thalassemics. The main principle is to eliminate the antigen derived from plasma protein and leukocytes and also platelets which may cause anaphylactic reaction.

Procedure

- Take out cross-matched blood bags with attached satellite bags.
- Start the refrigerated centrifuge machine before 30 minutes and adjust required temperature is 5°C at

1,500 RPM, ACCL 9 and DECL 5. RPM, TIME, ACCL and DECL can be changed according to needs because these parameters may differ from centrifuge to centrifuge (See Table 7.1).

- Carry out the whole procedure under the laminar airflow bench.
- Weight the blood bag bucket before centrifugation. Weight the opposite buckets should be equal.
- Before placing blood bag buckets inside the refrigerated centrifuge, check temperature of refrigerated centrifuge at 5°C.
- Place the blood bag buckets of the refrigerated centrifuge diagonally in opposite positions (Fig. 8.1).
- Keep the blood bag for centrifugation, i.e. 4,000 RPM, ACCL 9, and DECL 6 for 5 to 10 minutes at 5°C and remove plasma into satellite bag through plasma expresser. RPM, TIME, ACCL, and DECL can be changed according to needs because these parameters may differ from centrifuge to centrifuge (See Figs 7.1A and B).
- Double seal the tube between the pack cell bag and satellite bag, detach plasma bag from mother bag. Discard the plasma bag.
- Cold normal saline bottle (4°C) hang on saline stand; clean needle prick area of normal saline bottle and tubing area of mother bag by sterile spirit cotton with the help of sterile forceps under laminar airflow bench.
- Introduce 250 mL cold normal saline for 450 mL of blood and 150–200 mL normal saline for 350 mL of blood with the help of sterile disposable transfusion set to the pack cell bag.
- Seal the area of inserted needle by sealer and remove the needle from the tube of the bag and cover the needle with it in plastic cover.

- Mix well-packed cell with saline; place bucket and again weight by weight machine.
- Keep the bag for centrifugation at 'heavy spin', i.e. 4,000 RPM, ACCL 8, and DECL 5 for 10 minutes at 5°C. RPM, TIME, ACCL, and DECL can be changed according to needs because these parameters may differ from centrifuge to centrifuge (See Figs 7.1A and B and Table 7.1).
- After centrifugation remove the bag carefully and express the supernatant into transfer port.
- Repeat this process three times.
- After final wash add 50–60 mL of saline into packed cell and mix.
- Seal the bag with the help of sealer machine.
- Allow it for issue as soon as possible. If delayed transfusion should be stored at 2–6°C temperature not more than 24 hours.

Chapter 9

Preservation and Distribution of Blood Components

Storage of Blood Components

- Whole blood and packed cells (SAGM-2/ADSOL preservative) should be stored at 2–6°C temperature in blood bank refrigerator (See Fig.15.1).
- FFP/Cryopoor Plasma and platelet-poor plasma should be stored at (–80°C to –40°C) deep frozen for 24 hours. After solidification transfer plasma bag to chamber chest deep freeze at –30°C till expiry date. Keep it in plastic packets (See Figs 8.3A and B).
- For cryoprecipitate component blast freeze at –80°C temperature is very effective because it gets rapid freezing and amount of factor VIII is more available in cryoprecipitate component (See Fig. 8.4).
- Platelets concentrate is kept at 22–24°C in platelet agitator incubator after 1 hour interval. Plain surface area of the bag should always be kept on upper side in agitator and label area should keep down side in the agitator. Because platelets bag have many pores which provide scope to supply oxygen for survival of platelets (See Figs 8.5A and B).
- Always keep single bag in the area. Do not overlap the bags.
- Agitate the agitator for (stroke) 70–72/minutes.

Thawing Procedure

- Before thawing of FFP and cryoprecipitate component, cryowater bath temperature should maintain according to needs and during thawing component bags should be kept inside plastic packet.

FFP

Before thawing FFP components, switch on cryowater bath and maintain at 37°C temperature (See Fig.7.3).

- Component thaw in circulating cryowater bath at 37°C within 30–45 minutes and it should not thaw at room temperature or running tap water, because stable and unstable coagulation factors will decrease.
- If thawed in a water bath, the entry ports must be protected so that water cannot contaminate the units.
- An approved microwave thawing device can thaw FFP component at the temperature of 37°C (Sally V. Rudmann, page 247, 2nd edition).
- After thawing, issue FFP component product immediately specially for correction of unstable clotting factors. If issue is delayed then keep at 4°C and it should be used within 6 hours. It cannot be refrozen after thawing.

Cryoprecipitate

- Before thawing cryoprecipitate component circulating cryowater bath temperature should be maintained at 4°C (See Fig. 7.3).
- Cryo will thaw at 4°C cold room or blood bank refrigerator. It should also thaw in circulating cryowater bath within 30– 45 minutes.
- During thawing put cryo with cryo bag inside the circulating cryowater bath and hang satellite bag (cryopoor plasma collection) at outside of the water bath. It will thaw upto 30–45 minutes.
- After centrifugation transferring cryopoor plasma into

satellite bag and white flakes will be visible in cryo bag. This bag (cryo bag) can be stored again at −80°C or lower for 1 year and after thawing at 4°C and it can be used.
- White flakes will dissolve in short period at 25–30°C within 5–10 minutes.
- White flakes is labile factor, it should mix gently by hand and dissolve automatically within few minutes. Allow for transfusion immediately (This process is better because reducing chance of factor VIII is less).
• White flakes factor VIII will be active for short duration, once thawed it should issue within 6 hours. Before issue, cryo bag kept at 4°C blood bank refrigerator.

Cryopoor plasma

Thawing procedure should be same as FFP component procedure (See Fig. 7.3).

Platelet-poor plasma

Thawing procedure should be same as FFP component procedure (See Fig. 7.3).

Procedure to Issue Components

- Blood grouping must be confirmed before issue (by reverse method).
- Cross-match with recipient cells must be done before issue.
- Antibody screening test must be done using Coombs reagent and pooled 'O' cells.
  - Before issue check all records of mandatory test like HIV 1–2, HBsAg, anti-HCV, VDRL and MP. It should be (nonreactive).

- Before issue check record register and computer records.
- Component product showing any hemolysis or bacterial contamination should not be issued.
- Before issue check the bag whether it has a leakage or damage.
- For platelets concentrate, swirling phenomenon should be checked before. There should be no grossly visible platelet aggregates during the storage.
- Platelets and cryo component should be administered through special standard filter (170 micron). Micro aggregate filters should not be used for these products.

Chapter 10

Component Transfusion's Dose and Rate of Infusion

Fresh Frozen Plasma

Volume of 1 unit fresh frozen plasma (FFP) is 200–250 mL (prepared from 450 mL of whole blood). Appropriate dose is 10–15 mL/kg of body weight. It contains 1 IU/mL of each coagulation factors and fibrinogen 200–400 mg (See Fig. 8.2B).

Indication of FFP

FFP is used in patients with bleeding due to multiple coagulation factor deficiencies, such as in liver disease, disseminated intravascular coagulation (DIC) and dilutional coagulopathy, thrombotic thrombocytopenic purpura (TTP), familial deficiency of factor-V, deficiency of factors II, VII, IX, antithormbin-III.

Moreover the transfusion of FFP in conjunction with packed RBC replaced the maximum demands of fresh blood.

- **Monitoring of FFP transfusion**—Post-transfusion determination of APTT and PT.
- **When to transfusion**—Thawed plasma should be transfused as early as possible. If transfusion may be delayed, it must be transfused within 12 hours (preferably 6 hours) in that case it must be stored at 2–4°C.
- **Cross-matching**—FFP should be ABO compatible with patients blood. Precaution must be taken that donors

should not contain ABO antibodies that may cross react with A or B antigen on recipients RBC. Rh-compatible FFP to be given (but Rh-positive plasma should not be given to Rh-negative women in reproductive age group).

- **Contraindication**:
  - **Contraindications FFP transfusion**—Contraindications of FFP transfusion with normal PT. For replenishing the blood volume, management of hypoproteinemia or as source of immunoglobulin.
  - **Result of FFP transfusion**—After transfusion of 1 unit of FFP the coagulation factors may be raised 2–3%. How to prevent the loss of FFP, if transfused in pediatrics—FFP can be prepared by dividing in lesser volume before freezing, average 60 mL/units.
- **Side effects**:
1. Acute allergic reactions are common.
2. Febrile, nonhemolytic reaction.
3. Viral transmission.
4. Bacterial contamination—Sepsis.
5. Rarely TRALI (transmitted-related acute lung infection).

Platelets Concentrate

- The usual adult dose is 4–6 units of random donor platelets (1 unit/10 kg). Transfusion medicine consultation is advised concerning the exact dose. In pediatrics patient the usual platelets dose is 5 mL/kg of body weight. The standard administration set with 170 micron filter may be used. In general platelets are given as quickly as possible.
- 1 unit of platelets 50–60 mL.
  Calculation of rise of platelet—1 unit of random donors platelet increases the platelet count by

5,000–10,000/cmm whereas 1 unit of apheresis platelet increases platelet count by 30,000–60,000/cmm.

- Calculation of platelet required.
  Blood Volume (BV) – rough calculation 70 mL/kg body weight /other method $2.5 \times$ body surface (m^2).
  PL—Desired platelet count increment
  0.67 = dose normally recoverable
  Formula of platelet required—BV × PL/0.67.

  Monitoring of patient response to platelet transfusion—Perform platelet count post-transfusion at 10 minute, 15 minutes, 1 hour or 20 hours.

- **Complications**: Fever, chill, allergic reaction are common in patients receiving multiple transfusions. In addition transmission of viral hepatitis, development of resistant state, graft versus host disease (GVHD) may develop. Immunization against RBC may occur if platelet concentrate is contaminated with RBC.

Cryoprecipitate

Each bag contain 15–20 mL plasma.

Cryoprecipitate contains—Factor VIII, fibrinogen. von Willebrand factor, fibronectin, factor XIII.

- **Cryoprecipitate is indicated in**
  - Hemophilia.
  - von Willebrand disease.
  - DIC.
  - In some condition of acute leukemia.
  - Hypofibrinogenemia.
  - Deficiency of factor XIII and acquired deficiency of factor VIII.
  - In premature neonate platelet count less than 50000/cmm.

- Platelet count less than 100000/cmm in distressed infants.
- **Contraindications**: Specific factor deficiency which is not present in cryoprecipitate.
- **Side effects**: Very rarely viral hepatitis, commonly fever, allergic.
- **Mode of issue**: Cryoprecipitate preferably given ABO matching but it is not mandatory.
- **Dose**: The number of cryoprecipitate units can be estimated by using the following calculation:

    Blood volume (mL) of patient = Weight (kg) × 70 mL/kg; Plasma volume (mL) = Blood volume (mL) × (1.0-hematocrit); Fibrinogen required (mg) = [Target fibrinogen (mg/dL) − initial fibrinogen (mg/dL)] × plasma volume (mL) ÷ 100.

    Bags of cryo required = Fibrinogen (mg) required ÷ 150 mg fibrinogen per bag.

Calculation for factor VIII

1 IU of factor VIII/kg body weight will increase Factor VIII 2% half-life 12 hours so, factor VIII transfusion to be repeated 8–12 hours.

In case of major surgery factor VIII should be maintained 40% for at least 10 days.

Monitoring–PTT is the rough guide for factor VIII activity. PTT normal indicates factor VIII is at least 30%.
Units of factor VIII desired = (desired factor VIII level in units/mL − initial level of factor VIII/mL) × plasma volume in mL.

1971- HBsAg antigen testing introduced for safe blood transfusion

1981 – First AIDS case reported and from 1985 – screening of HIV in donated blood started. From 1998 – Hepatitis C testing became mandatory for blood transfusion

Infusion Rates of Various Components

Block

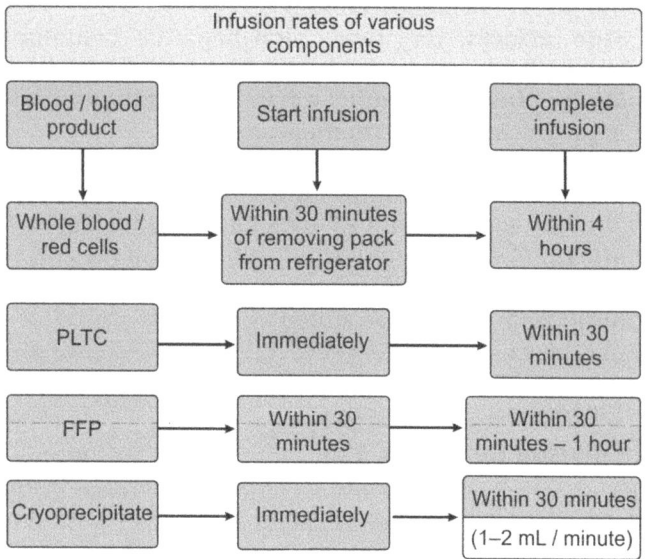

* Rate of infusion of whole blood or PRBC, FFP, platelets concentrate and cryoprecipitate component depends on patients' clinical condition.

* Before infusion of platelets concentrate components must be shaken gently by hand.

Chapter 11

Quality Control

Sterility Tests

- **Material**:
  - Specimen
  - Incubator to maintain 37°C
  - Culture media
  - For gram-positive:
    1. Nutrient agar
    2. MacConkey's agar
    3. Blood agar
    4. Chocolate agar
  - For gram-negative:
    1. MacConkey's agar
    2. Nutrient broth
  - For subcultures:
    1. Tungsten wire-loop/platinum wire loop
    2. Bunsen's burner
    3. Culture plates (covered Petri dishes).

- **Methods**:
  - Heat wire loop till red hot.
  - Cool.
  - Take one loopful of specimen.
  - Inoculate culture plate with wire loop with streak method.

- Incubate for 36–48 hours in:
  a. Nutrient agar
  b. McLeod's agar
  c. Blood agar.
- Examine for growth.
- Examine growth and specimen both for bacterium by Gram's staining.

Quality Control Specifications and Procedures for Blood Components

The Quality Control of Whole Blood (Table 11.1)

- ☐ **Volume**: Weight at least 1% of donations and calculated the volume from the formula given below.
- Vol (mL) = Weight of bag + blood(gm) – weight of empty bag (gm).

Table 11.1: Quality control of whole blood

Parameter	Quality requirement
Volume	350 mL/450 mL +/– 10%
Anticoagulants*	49 mL/63 mL
PCV (Hct)	30–40%
HBsAg	Negative by ELISA
Anti-HCV	Negative by ELISA
Syphilis	Negative by screening test
Sterility	By culture

Note: * Volume of anticoagulant should be proportionate to the volume of blood. 14 mL of CPD/ CPDA-1 anticoagulant solutions is required for 100 mL of blood.

* Drugs controller general INDIA, NBTC.

Red Cell Concentration

- Free from bacterial contamination.
- Red cell concentration should pass all mandatory tests, that are HIV, HBsAg, HCV, VDRL, and malaria parasites.
- Hematocrit: 75% to 80% in packed cells and SAGM-2 preservative packed cell 60%.
- Specific gravity 1.09.
- Volume 250 mL ± 10% when processed for 450 mL bag.

Saline-washed Packed Cells (Leuko Reduce Poor Red Cells)

- If prepared by centrifugation 70% of WBC's should be removed and 70% of RBC's of the original quality retained.
- Leukocyte counts on pre and postwashed packed cells should be done. Yield of WBC $<1 \times 10^9$ cells/unit of washed cells.
- Bag should be checked for hemolysis.
- Bacteriological culture should be done if suspected.

Platelet Concentrate by Platelet-rich Plasma

- Volume: 50–60 mL.
- $P^H > 6.0$.
- Platelet count from 450 mL whole blood should $> 4.5 \times 10^{10}$/unit and 350 mL whole blood $> 3.5 \times 10^{10}$/unit (it also depends on platelet count of the individual area).
- RBC contamination 0.5 mL and WBC contamination $5.5 \times 10^7 - 5 \times 10^5$.
- Free from bacterial contamination.

Platelet Concentrate by Buffy-coat with Plasma

- Volume: 70–90 mL
- Platelet count 6 to 9×10^{10}

- $P^H > 6.0$
- WBC contamination $> 5.5 \times 10^6$
- RBC contamination trace to 0.5 mL
- Free from bacterial contamination.

Precautions to be Taken while Sampling for Quality Check

- Adequate mixing.
- Samples for Hb/platelet count should be taken into a dry EDTA tube.

Quality control checked for platelets count:

1. Mixing of product and proper stripping of tubing so that sample represents the actual product. Bag tubing containing the sample may be detached using an electric sealer. This practice preserves the original bag and prevents platelet shortage.
- Sampling methods must be validated to ensure that they produce consistent samples, regardless of the operator.
2. As the life of the platelets is 5 days, so we need to check platelets concentrate for each and every bag, but in practice we sample out few bags randomly and check the platelet concentration by standard procedure like platelets count analyzer or platelets counting chamber.
- Platelet recovery in vivo influenced by freshness of platelets, 10% decrease in the recovery with every 24 hours storage. Recovery is also affected by the antiplatelet antibodies like PLA anticipated platelet increment, i.e. API, after transfusion should be calculated as followed.
- $$API = \frac{\text{Total no. of platelet transfused}}{\text{Blood volume/Body weight in gm}} \times 2/3$$
- Platelets yield = platelet/mm^3 × 1000 × vol of platelet. in mL.

Fresh Frozen Plasma (FFP)

- Plasma should be separated from whole blood within 6–8 hours of collection (preferably 6 hours).
- Volume of FFP 200–250 mL, depending upon whether the blood bag is supplied with SAGM-2 or not.
- Stable coagulation factors: 200 units.
- Factor VIII: 0.7 IU/mL.
- Fibrinogen: 200–400 mg.

Cryoprecipitate: (Factor VIII)

- Volume: 15–20 mL/unit.
- Factor VIII: 80–120 IU.
- Fibrinogen: 150–250 mg.
- von Willebrand factor (vWF): 40–70% of the original.
- Factor XIII: 20–30% of the original.
- Factor II, V, IX: Small fraction.
- Fibronectin: 55 mg.

Additional Quality Control Things

- All components labels are waterproof.
- Components are not released to stock unless the mandatory tests reports are available.
- The components are stored at the proper temperature with continuous recording of the temperature.
- Temperature of waterbath and incubators should be checked on daily basis.
- Calibration is done for proper speed of centrifuge.
- Temperature of deep freezer should be checked on daily basis.

Chapter 12

Biomedical Waste Management

Biomedical Waste

All human activities produce waste. We all know that such waste may be dangerous and needs safe disposal. Industrial waste, sewage, and agricultural waste pollute water, soil, and air. It can also be dangerous to human beings and environment. Similarly, hospitals and other health care facilities generate lots of waste which can transmit infections, particularly HIV, hepatitis B, hepatitis C, and tetanus, to the people who handle it or come in contact with it.

Most countries of the world, specially the developing nations, are facing the grim situation arising out of environmental pollution due to pathological waste arising from increasing population and the consequent rapid growth in the number of health care centers. India is no exception to this and it is estimated that there are more than 15,000 small and private hospitals and nursing homes in the country. This is apart from clinics and pathological labs, which also generate sizeable amounts of medical waste.

India generates around three million tonnes of medical wastes every year and the amount is expected to grow at 8% annually. Creating large dumping grounds and incinerators is the first step and some progressive states such as Maharashtra, Karnataka, and Tamil Nadu are making efforts despite opposition.

☐ **Definition**: Any waste which is generated during the diagnosis, treatment or immunization of human beings or animals or in research or in production or testing of biological is called biomedical waste.

The rule of biomedical waste is prescribed by the Ministry of Environment and Forest, Government of India and applied on 28th July 1998 to those who generate, collect, receive, stor, dispose, treat or handle the source in however.

Biomedical Waste Consists of

- Human anatomical wastes like tissues, organs, and body parts.
- Animal wastes generated during research from veterinary hospitals.
- Microbiology and biotechnology wastes.
- Waste sharps like hypodermic needles, syringes, scalpels, and broken glasses.
- Discarded medicines and cytotoxic drugs.
- Soiled wastes such as dressings, bandages, plaster casts, material contaminated with blood, tubes, and catheters.
- Liquid wastes from any of the infected areas.
- Incineration ashes and other chemical wastes.

Methods of Disposal

1. Incineration
2. Chemical disinfection
3. Autoclaving
4. Microwave irradiation
5. Controlled tripping/sanitary landfill/deep burial.

Biomedical Waste Management in Relation to Blood Banking Activities

Biomedical wastes should be segregated into color-coded containers and bags as laid down in the rule, at the point of generation of wastes. Details of which is shown in the Table 12.1.

Table 12.1: Biomedical waste management

	Treatment	Packing	Final disposal transportation
Glass tubes	Soak in 1% sodium hypochlorite solution for 1 hour	Transparent plastic bag	In white transparent plastic bag
Blood bags, swab, soiled cotton	Autoclave	Yellow bag	Yellow bucket
Patient sample tube (plastic)	Autoclave	Yellow bag	Yellow bucket
Blood bag segment	Autoclave	Blue bag	Blue bucket
Donor sample tube (plastic)	Soak in 1% sodium hypochlorite solution 1 hour	Blue bag	Blue bucket
Culture plate, tips, cards	Soak in 1% sodium hypochlorite solution 1 hour	Blue bag	Blue bucket
Disposable needle	Adjoining plastic segment	White container	White container

Contd...

Contd...

	Treatment	Packing	Final disposal transportation
	along with needle should be cut till the base of the needle. Destroy the needle, put the residue in the plastic puncture-proof translucent white container with 1% sodium hypochlorite solution		
Glass slides, sharp	After soaking in 1% sodium hypochlorite solution, materials should be kept in white translucent puncture-proof container	White container	White container

- Buckets meant for keeping the waste material like culture plates, cotton, swabs, needles, slides, etc. should be filled with 1% sodium hypochlorite solution.
- After proper treatment and segregation, the material should be sent for incineration.
- Always wear gloves while handling blood specimens.

- Follow the instructions of biomedical waste at every section of the blood bank.

Preparation of Sodium Hypochlorite Solution

Available chlorine (Labeled on bottle)	To prepare 0.1% sodium hypochlorite solution	To prepare 1% sodium hypochlorite solution
Sodium hypochlorite (Available chlorine 4%)	2.5 mL sodium hypochlorite + 97.5 mL distil water	25 mL sodium hypochlorite+75 mL distil water
Sodium hypochlorite (Available chlorine 5%)	2.0 mL sodium hypochlorite + 98.0 mL distil water	20 mL sodium hypochlorite + 80 mL distil water

- Sodium hypochlorite solution with a concentration of 0.1% available chlorine is used for wiping work benches specimen containers, etc.
- A stronger solution with concentration of 1% available chlorine is used for disinfecting blood spillage and heavily contaminated equipments.
- Sodium hypochlorite solutions gradually lose their strength. Require daily preparation.

Disinfection Protocol

Chapter 13

Procedure

Step I

Blood bags, fresh frozen plasma (FFP) bags, platelet concentrates (PLTC) bags, and cryoprecipitate bags that require to be discarded should be autoclaved at the specified temperature for the specified time at 121°C and 15 pound pressure for 30 minutes with biological indicator. After autoclaving check the biological indicator. If color is changed, it indicates these bags are properly disinfected and then can be discarded into yellow bags to be sent for incineration.

Step II

In general blood banking practice blood bags and other respective components bag like FFP, PLTC and cryoprecipitate, etc. that require to be discarded should be injected with 20 mL of 4% sodium hypochlorite solution by disposable syringes through connecting satellite tubes very carefully.

After completion injected area should be sealed by selar machine. After that mix it properly and wait for

30 minutes. Then follow above-mentioned remaining steps. During this process gloves should be worn (See Fig. 14.1).

Method for preparation: 1% bleaching powder solution
- Take 10 liter of water (one bucket)
- Take 100 gm or one matchbox full of bleaching powder
- Mix it properly

A well-known complication of early blood transfusion was transmission of syphilis–one factor which led to the routine serological screening of blood donor for syphilis.

Later on Australia Ag. For hepatitis B, and in 1980's HIV. Nowadays screening for 5 diseases (HBV, HCV, HIV, malaria, and syphilis) is mandatory in blood transfusion service

Chapter 14

Sterilization

Autoclave (Sterilizer) (Fig. 14.1)

- **Purpose**: It is one of the important equipment of Operating Room Equipment without which any operation is impossible. With the help of this equipment sterilization is done for killing the fungi, bacteria, and viruses.

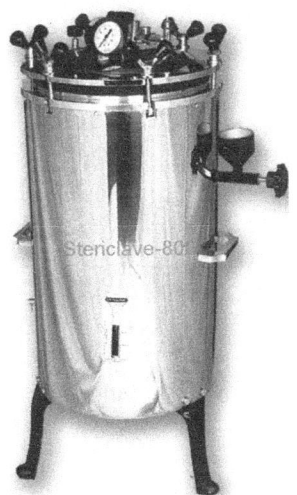

Figure 14.1: Autoclave (sterilizer)

This sterilization is also applied to linen, clothes, objects, and tools. There are several methods of sterilization such as steam heating, dry heating, ethylene oxide gas method, cold sterilization by cidex, automatic decontamination system (cidematic) and radiation technique.

- **Principle**: From the several methods of sterilization, the steam sterilization is mostly used and the simplest sterilization equipment is called 'Autoclave' and is of two types:
  a. Vertical type
  b. Horizontal type.

1. Vacuum period: The air of the inner chamber is withdrawn.
2. Steam storing period: In the outside chamber which is made of 304 graded stainless steel allows the super heated steam to enter from boiler. The pressure and temperature of inner chamber is raised by 20 psi and 120°C.
3. Sterilization period: The super heated steam enters in the inner chamber where the material is stored. When the inner chamber's temperature is 120°C and pressure is 20 psi, the sterilization starts. As per sterilization norm this stage is kept for 20 minutes. All the bacteria inside the chamber are killed in this condition. A special type of indicator which is rapped on the material before sterilization, changes the color.
4. Exhaust period: After 20 minutes of operation the steam present in the inner chamber is allowed to exhaust outside from the chamber and the pressure falls to zero.
5. Drying period: After the exhaust period, the inner chamber is kept into vacuum line for the residual steam to come out and then the sterilized item

becomes dry. The above process is done with multiport valve which is made up to Gun Metal. Autoclaves have two chambers for boiler to produce steam and another one for sterilization. With the help of electric heater or gas burner steam can be generated.

Chapter 15

Blood Bank Refrigerator

- **Purpose**: The blood should be stored at a temperature of 4°C (±2°C). It would be damaged and cannot be used

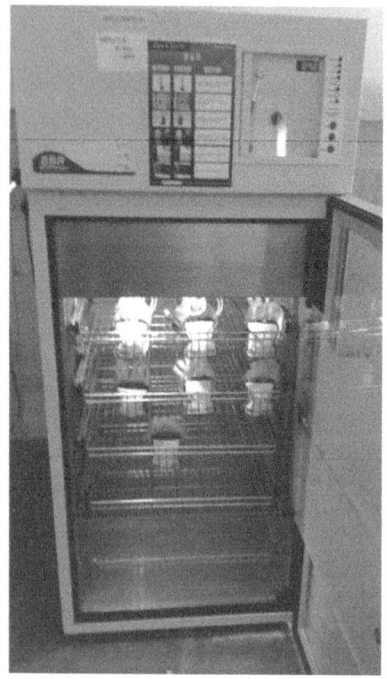

Figure 15.1: Blood bank refrigerator

above or below this temperature. So we must need the blood bank refrigerator to keep the whole blood (Fig. 15.1; See Plate 5 for color figure).

- **Principle**: The refrigerator used by blood bank has two chambers that are inner and outer chambers. Between the two chambers, the glass wool is laminated to prevent temperature of outside to move in. The freon gas is highly compressed and allows expanding in the cooling chamber (by Joule-Thompson effect). The temperature of the inner chamber is made uniform with the help of a blower fan. Temperature controller measured and compared the temperature of the chamber with set point. If the temperature is low than the set point, the controller start the compressor to make temperature high. The temperature sensor which is set in inner chamber will provide signal to the controller to control display and record the temperature.

- **Block Diagram**:

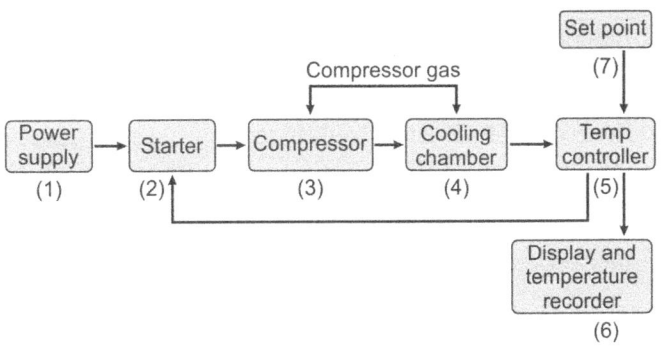

1. Provide power to the starter.
2. Starter will start or off the control as per received signal from the temperature controller.
3. Compressor delivered the compressed gas to the cooling chamber and also collect the noncompressed gas from cooling chamber.

4. Cooling chamber, here the compressed gas goes to an adiabatic expansion and temperature fall.
5. Temperature controller receives the signal from sensor and advice starter to start or off the compressor.
6. The temperature of the inner chamber is displayed and recorded on the graph.
7. It is a device by which the temperature can be set at desired value.

- **Job Chart**:
1. Power supply to be checked
2. Earthing to be checked
3. Proper cooling is made or not
4. Proper door locking is made or not
5. Inside lamp blows or not.

- **Trouble Shooting**:
1. No cooling.
   Remedy—Compressor to be checked.
2. No display of temperature.
   Remedy—Display board circuit is to be checked.
3. Abnormal sound after starting.
   Remedy—Mechanical fouling to be checked.
4. Temperature graph may not rotate.
   Remedy—Motor driven system to be checked.

> Always keep packed cells blood in horizontal position and also keep whole blood in vertical position (blood bank refrigerator) at 2–6°C temperature

Further Reading

1. AABB Misconceptions about TRALI risk, reduction recommendations.
2. American cancer society. aabb.org. American Redcross.
3. Bercher ME (Ed). Technical Manual 15th ed. Bethesda: American Association of Blood Banks. 2005.
4. Bharucha Z, Chouhan DM, Model Standard Operating Procedures for Blood Transfusion Service (WHO, New Delhi). 1st edition. 1990; 12/16.
5. Blood Transfusion: A basic text publication by WHO edition 2004 (History of Blood Banking).
6. Component Preparation Guidelines standards for Blood banks and Blood transfusion services, NACO (NBTC). 2007.
7. Drugs Controller General, INDIA (NBTC).
8. Biomedical waste—Bailley, Redcross society.
9. Gernsheimer T. Blood component therapy. Puget Sound Blood Centre Transfusion Services. 2010.
10. Guidelines for requisition, handling, storage and transfusion of blood and blood components, department of Transfusion Medicine AIIMS, New Delhi.
11. Guide to the preparation, use and quality assurance of blood components, 7th edition. Council of Europe Publishing. 1998.
12. Harmening DM (Ed). Modern blood banking and transfusion practices, 4th ed. Philadelphia: FA Davis Company. 1999.
13. Malik V. Drugs and Cosmetics Act of India. 2001.
14. Mollison PL, Engelfriet CP, Contreras M. Blood transfusion in clinical medicine 10th ed. Oxford Blackwell Science Ltd. 1998.
15. Park K A textbook of preventive and social medicine, 12th ed. 2013.
16. Rudmann VS textbook of blood banking and transfusion medicine 2nd ed.

17. Sankalp India Foundation, under the management of Indian Blood Bank Society.
18. Simon TL, Dzik WH, Synder EL, Stowell CP, Strauss RG, (Eds). Rossi's Principles of Transfusion Medicine. Lippincott. Williams and Wilkins Publication.

Index

A

ABO blood group systems 24
Additional quality control things 107

B

Bag selection 25
Basic informations for blood components product 37
Benefits and advantages of blood components 7
Biomedical waste management 108, 110
    in relation to blood banking activities 110
Blood bags buckets 34
Blood bank refrigerator 118
    block diagram 119
    job chart 120
    principle 119
    purpose 118
    trouble shooting 120
Blood collection techniques for donor
    phlebotomy procedure 11
Blood components preparation by quadruple bags 83, 87
Blood components 3
    functions of
        plasma 3
        platelets 4
        RBC 3
        WBC 3
    preservation and distribution 94
    separation 5
Blood group choice
    for PLTC 22
    for PRBC and whole blood 21
Buckets 42

C

Calculation for factor VIII 101
Care after donation 15
Check calibration of cryofuge centrifuge 6000i and other models of refrigerated centrifuge 48
    RPM 49
    temperature 48
Circulating plasma/cryowater bath 54
Common blood type in Indian people 24
Common things to be done
    before preparation of blood components 31
    during preparation of blood components 35
Component transfusion's dose and rate of infusion 98
Cryopoor plasma 96
Cryoprecipitate 9, 32, 95, 100
    contraindications 101
    dose 101
    mode of issue 101
    side effects 101
Cryoprecipitate component preparation 66, 82
    by hanging method 68
    from FFP bag 38

D

Defer the donor temporarily 18
Disinfection protocol procedure 113
Donor selection 10

E

Electronic sealer operation of 55
Equipments and materials required for components preparation 28

F

FFP component for pediatric patient 36
Fresh frozen plasma (FFP) 8, 32, 98, 107
  contraindication 99
  indication 98
  side effects 99

G

General awareness and precaution for donor 14

H

Handling of
  circulating plasma/cryowater bath 55
  cryofuge centrifuge 6000i and other models of refrigerated centrifuge 46
Health benefits of donating blood
  reduce the chance of heart diseases 17
Horizontal laminar airflow bench 53

I

Infusion rates of various components 102
Instruction followed for blood components preparation 37
Instruction follows after preparation of platelet concentrate in triple bags and quadruple bags 74

L

Leuko-depleted packed cell, FFP and cryoprecipitate components preparation 78
Leuko-depleted packed cell/fresh frozen plasma by triple bags collection 63

M

Materials required for blood components product 41
Methodology of blood components preparation 10
Methods of disposal 109
Modern transfusion medicine 7

N

Neutral plasma 8

P

Packed red blood cell/leuko-depleted packed cell and saline-washed packed red cell 8

Index

Packed red blood cell (leuko-depleted)/platelets concentrate by (PRP method) and platelet-poor plasma (PPP/ FFP) in quadruple bags 84

Packed red blood cell (PRBC)/cryoprecipitate/cryo-poor plasma by triple bags collection 65

Packed red blood cell (PRBC)/fresh frozen plasma (FFP) by double bags collection 58
   materials required 58

Packed red blood cell (PRBC)/platelets concentrate/platelets-poor plasma (fresh frozen plasma (PPP/FFP) by random donor in triple bags collection 69

Packed red blood cells (leuko-depleted), fresh frozen plasma/cryoprecipitate by quadruple bags (SAGM-2/adsol preservative) 81

Packed red blood cell (leuko-depleted/ platelets concentrate by (PRP method) and platelet-poor plasma (PPP/FFP) in quadruple bags 84

Packed red blood cell (PRBC)/platelets concentrate by (PRP method)/platelet-poor plasma (PPP/FFP)/cryoprecipitate or required amount of FFP for pediatrics patient in quadruple bags 87

Packed red blood (PRBC) cell (leuko-depleted)/platelets concentrate by (buffy-coat method)/FFP preparation in quadruple bags 71

Platelets concentrate 9, 99
   by buffy-coat with plasma 105
   by platelet-rich plasma 105

Platelet-poor plasma 96

Platelet-rich plasma (PRP) 9

Precautions 28
   required for blood components preparation 30
   required for blood components preparation area 28
   to be taken while sampling for quality check 106

Preparation of
   blood components—procedures 57
   leuko-depleted packed cells 80
   sodium hypochlorite solution 112

Procedure to issue components 96

Programing of cryofuge 6000i 45

Q

Quality control 103
   of whole blood 104
      specifications and procedures for blood components 104

R

Red cell concentration 105
Refrigerated centrifuge 45
Restricted person for blood donation 19

S

Safe handling of equipments 44
Safe plasma transfusion 24
Saline-washed packed cells (leuko reduce poor red cells) 105
Saline-washed packed red blood cells (PRBC) in double bags preparation (450 mL/350 mL)
   material required 90
   principle 91
   procedure 91
Sterility tests
   material 103
   methods 103
Sterilization
   autoclave 115
Storage of blood components 94

T

Thawing procedure 94
Transfusion transmitted infection (TTI) 20

W

Weighing scale 36